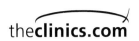

Agnes E. Rupley, DVM, Dipl. ABVP–Avian
CONSULTING EDITOR

VETERINARY CLINICS

OF NORTH AMERICA

Exotic Animal Practice

Hematology and Related Disorders

GUEST EDITOR
Tarah L. Hadley, DVM, Dipl. ABVP–Avian

September 2008 • Volume 11 • Number 3

SAUNDERS

An Imprint of Elsevier, Inc.
PHILADELPHIA   LONDON   TORONTO   MONTREAL   SYDNEY   TOKYO

W.B. SAUNDERS COMPANY

A Division of Elsevier Inc.

1600 John F. Kennedy Blvd., Suite 1800, Philadelphia, PA 19103-2899

http://www.vetexotic.theclinics.com

VETERINARY CLINICS OF NORTH AMERICA:	Volume 11, Number 3
EXOTIC ANIMAL PRACTICE	ISSN 1094-9194
September 2008	ISBN-13: 978-1-4160-6370-4
Editor: John Vassallo; j.vassallo@elsevier.com	ISBN-10: 1-4160-6370-6

Veterinary Clinics of North America: Exotic Animal Practice (ISSN 1094-9194) is published in January, May, and September by Elsevier, Inc.; Business and Editorial offices: 1600 John F. Kennedy Blvd., Suite 1800, Philadelphia, PA 19103-2899. Customer Service Office: 6277 Sea Harbor Drive, Orlando, FL 32887-4800. Subscription prices are $161.00 per year for US individuals, $288.00 per year for US institutions, $84.00 per year for US students and residents, $190.00 per year for Canadian individuals, $333.00 per year for Canadian institutions, $202.00 per year for international individuals, $333.00 per year for international institutions and $101.00 per year for Canadian and foreign students/residents. To receive student/resident rate, orders must be accompanied by name of affiliated institution, date of term, and the *signature* of program/residency coordinator on institution letterhead. Orders will be billed at individual rate until proof of status is received. Foreign air speed delivery is included in all *Clinics* subscription prices. All prices are subject to change without notice.

POSTMASTER: Send address changes to *Veterinary Clinics of North America: Exotic Animal Practice*; Elsevier Periodicals Customer Service, 6277 Sea Harbor Drive, Orlando, FL 32887-4800. **Customer Service: 1-800-654-2452 (US). From outside of the United States, call 1-407-563-6020. Fax: 1-407-363-9661. E-mail: JournalsCustomer Service-usa@elsevier.com.**

Reprints. For copies of 100 or more of articles in this publication, please contact the commercial Reprints Department, Elsevier Inc., 360 Park Avenue South, New York, New York 10010-1710. Tel: (212) 633-3813 Fax: (212) 633-1935, e-mail: reprints@elsevier.com.

Veterinary Clinics of North America: Exotic Animal Practice is covered in *MEDLINE/PubMed (Index Medicus)*.

Printed in the United States of America.

CONSULTING EDITOR

AGNES E. RUPLEY, DVM, Diplomate, American Board of Veterinary Practitioners–Avian; Director and Chief Veterinarian, All Pets Medical & Laser Surgical Center, College Station, Texas

GUEST EDITOR

TARAH L. HADLEY, DVM, Diplomate, American Board of Veterinary Practitioners– Avian; Atlanta Hospital for Birds and Exotics, Inc., Conyers, Georgia

CONTRIBUTORS

MATTHEW C. ALLENDER, DVM, MS, Resident in Zoological Medicine, Department of Small Animal Clinical Sciences, College of Veterinary Medicine, University of Tennessee, Knoxville, Tennessee

JILL E. ARNOLD, MS, MT, National Aquarium in Baltimore, Baltimore, Maryland

ERIKA L. CERVASIO, DVM, Staff Veterinarian, Ocean State Veterinary Specialists, East Greenwich, Rhode Island

SHERRIE G. CLARK, DVM, MS, PhD, Diplomate, American College of Theriogenology; Assistant Professor, Department of Veterinary Clinical Medicine, University of Illinois at Urbana-Champaign, Illinois

TONYA M. CLAUSS, DVM, MS, Veterinary Services and Conservation Medicine, Georgia Aquarium, Atlanta, Georgia

NATALIE COFFER, BVetMed, MS, Diplomate, American College of Veterinary Internal Medicine; Visiting Clinical Assistant Professor, Department of Veterinary Clinical Medicine, University of Illinois at Urbana-Champaign, Illinois

ALISTAIR D.M. DOVE, PhD, Veterinary Services and Conservation Medicine, Georgia Aquarium, Atlanta, Georgia

STEPHEN M. DYER, DVM, Diplomate, American Board of Veterinary Practitioners– Avian; Staff Veterinarian, VCA South Shore Animal Hospital, Weymouth, Massachusetts

MICHAEL M. FRY, DVM, MS, Diplomate, American College of Veterinary Pathologists–Clinical Pathology; Assistant Professor, Department of Pathobiology, College of Veterinary Medicine, University of Tennessee, Knoxville, Tennessee

JENNIFER JOHNS, DVM, Diplomate, American College of Veterinary Pathologists–Clinical Pathology; PhD Student, Graduate Group of Comparative Pathology, Department of Pathology, Microbiology, and Immunology, School of Veterinary Medicine, University of California-Davis, Davis, California

STEPHEN A. KANIA, MS, PhD, Associate Professor of Immunology and Infectious Diseases, Department of Comparative Medicine, College of Veterinary Medicine, University of Tennessee, Knoxville, Tennessee

ERIC KLAPHAKE, DVM, Diplomate, American College of Zoological Medicine, Diplomate, American Board of Veterinary Practitioners–Avian; Veterinarian, ZooMontana, Billings; and Veterinarian, Animal Medical Center, Bozeman, Montana

KEMBA L. MARSHALL, DVM, Diplomate, American Board of Veterinary Practitioners–Avian; Summertree Animal and Bird Clinic, Dallas, Texas

ELIZABETH B. MITCHELL, DVM, MA, Resident, Companion Avian and Exotic Pet Medicine, Veterinary Medical Teaching Hospital, University of California-Davis, Davis, California

ANTHONY A. PILNY, DVM, Diplomate, American Board of Veterinary Practitioners–Avian; Department Head, Avian and Exotic Pet Medicine, Animal Specialty Center, Yonkers, New York

LINDA J. SIPERSTEIN, DVM, VCA Wakefield Animal Hospital, Wakefield, Massachusetts

JOHN M. SYKES IV, DVM, Diplomate, American College of Zoological Medicine; Veterinarian, Gottlieb Animal Health and Conservation Center, Los Angeles Zoo, Los Angeles, California

CONTENTS

their hematologic parameters. Animals within this order have much diversity in size, anatomy, methods of restraint, and blood collection technique. Appropriate sample collection is often the most challenging aspect of the diagnostic protocol, and inappropriate restraint may cause a stress response that interferes with blood test results. For many of these patients, sedation is required and can also affect results as well. In most cases, however, obtaining a standard database is necessary and very possible when providing medical care for this popular group of pets.

Ferret Hematology and Related Disorders

Linda J. Siperstein

This article summarizes the general topic of ferret hematology, including discussion of restraint for phlebotomy and phlebotomy sites, red and white blood cell morphology, interpretation of the hemogram, and normal and abnormal factors affecting the hemogram. In addition, the apparent lack of blood groups and techniques for bone marrow aspirates and blood transfusion are addressed. There is much still to be learned about the ferret and its diseases. We often depend on tests as simple as the complete blood cell count to help guide us in our diagnosis and treatments of this patient.

Rabbit Hematology

Kemba L. Marshall

Using laboratory animal medicine as an established resource, companion animal veterinarians have access to many physiologic and basic science studies that we can now merge with our clinical impressions. By working with reference laboratories, companion animal veterinarians are poised to accelerate our knowledge of the normal rabbit rapidly. The aim of this article is to discuss normal hematopoiesis and infectious and metabolic diseases that specifically target the hemolymphatic system. Additionally, photographic representation of cell types is provided.

Normal Hematology and Hematologic Disorders in Potbellied Pigs

Sherrie G. Clark and Natalie Coffer

Potbellied pigs have become a notable portion of small animal and farm animal practitioners' caseload. Relatively little information is readily accessible for the veterinary practitioner in regard to normal hematologic values or alterations of the hemogram in response to disease, however. This article is a review of blood collection techniques in swine adaptable to potbellied pigs in addition to collection artifacts observed in the swine hemogram. Alterations of the hemogram in disease states that may be encountered in potbellied pig medicine are reviewed.

FORTHCOMING ISSUES

RECENT ISSUES

ELSEVIER
SAUNDERS

Vet Clin Exot Anim 11 (2008) xi–xii

VETERINARY
CLINICS
Exotic Animal Practice

Preface

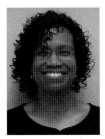

Tarah L. Hadley, DVM, DABVP–Avian
Guest Editor

I am honored to host this issue in the series on exotic animal practice. Beyond the initial physical examination, hematology is often one of the first diagnostic tools used by veterinarians to evaluate the medical status of healthy and ill animals. Many exotic animals are skilled at masking signs of illness from their caretakers. The need for a thorough understanding of this basic physiologic parameter is an essential first step in the medical evaluation process. I have brought together a diverse and dynamic group of contributors to explore the world of hematology in exotic animal species commonly seen in clinical practice. I thank all of them for their tireless efforts to make this issue relevant, updated, and informative.

This issue serves as an introduction to hematology for veterinarians who are new to the practice of exotic animal medicine. For the seasoned exotics veterinarian, this issue may offer some additional insight into previously explored areas, such as Dr. Stephen Kania's chapter on "Flow Cytometry Applications for Exotic Animals." I also encourage further exploration of the various textbooks, book chapters, and journal articles cited as references, which laid the foundation for this issue.

1094-9194/08/$ - see front matter © 2008 Elsevier Inc. All rights reserved.
doi:10.1016/j.cvex.2008.04.002   *vetexotic.theclinics.com*

I would like to dedicate this issue to one of my earliest mentors, Dr. Mark Pokras, Director of the Wildlife Clinic at Tufts University School of Veterinary Medicine. Enjoy!

Tarah L. Hadley, DVM, DABVP–Avian
Atlanta Hospital for Birds and Exotics, Inc.
2274 Salem Road, #106-149
Conyers, GA 30013, USA

E-mail address: drtarah@atlantabirdsandexotics.com

ELSEVIER
SAUNDERS

VETERINARY
CLINICS
Exotic Animal Practice

Vet Clin Exot Anim 11 (2008) 423–443

An Overview of Restraint and Blood Collection Techniques in Exotic Pet Practice

Stephen M. Dyer, DVM, DABVP–Avian[a],*,
Erika L. Cervasio, DVM[b]

[a]*VCA South Shore Animal Hospital, 595 Columbian Street, Weymouth, MA 02190, USA*
[b]*Ocean State Veterinary Specialists, 1480 South County Trail, East Greenwich, RI 02818, USA*

Blood sampling is considered part of the minimum database of any ill exotic pet. Even though interpretation of blood sample results is still in its infancy for many nontraditional pets, the diagnostic value of hematologic sampling will become greater with further research and clinical experience. In many exotic species, normal reference intervals are not available for even the most routine blood tests. Collecting blood samples from patients during wellness examinations helps define normal values for those individuals. The increased availability of biochemistry analyzers that sample small volumes of blood (VetScan, Abaxis, Union City, California) has made it possible to get many test results from pets that have only small volumes of blood to contribute. This article describes several techniques of obtaining and processing blood samples in a variety of nontraditional pets.

Tubes for blood collection

Because of the small size of many exotic patients, the volumes of blood that may be collected usually are very small. Blood collection tubes used for canine and feline patients often are too large to contain these samples, and the anticoagulant present causes significant dilution of the small sample. Instead, miniature container tubes (Microtainer, Becton-Dickinson, Franklin Lakes, New Jersey) designed for use in human pediatric medicine are ideal for handling small sample sizes common in exotic pet medicine. These

* Corresponding author.
E-mail address: sdyer@oregonducks.org (S.M. Dyer).

1094-9194/08/$ - see front matter © 2008 Elsevier Inc. All rights reserved.
doi:10.1016/j.cvex.2008.03.008   *vetexotic.theclinics.com*

tubes contain anticoagulant that is lyophilized (freeze-dried) so that sample dilution is not a problem.

The anticoagulants typically used include ethylenediaminetetraacetic acid (EDTA) and heparin. EDTA, found in lavender-top tubes, is a suitable anticoagulant for hematology testing and sample storage in most exotic pet patients. Exceptions to this include ostriches (Struthioniformes), crows (Corvidae), most reptiles, and many amphibians [1–4]. In these patients, the erythrocytes are susceptible to lysis in EDTA, so heparin, found in green-top tubes, should be used instead.

All anticoagulants can cause changes to erythrocytes that are apparent in a blood smear, either by altering the staining characteristics or by altering the size and shape of the cells themselves. Whenever possible, blood smears should be prepared at the time of blood draw, before they are exposed to anticoagulants [1]. In mammals, such as ferrets, rabbits, rodents, and marsupials, the smear may be prepared using two slides as in dog and cat samples. This slide-to-slide technique often is too harsh for the fragile erythrocytes of avian, amphibian, and reptile species, causing many of the cells to rupture [1]. A second technique, using a long coverslip (22 mm × 40 mm) on a slide, reduces the number of ruptured cells. A small drop of blood is placed on the slide and the long coverslip is placed on top of this at 90° to the slide. The coverslip then is slid past the slide to create the smear. A third technique involves using two square coverslips (22 mm × 22 mm). This last technique may provide the best smear with the fewest number of ruptured cells [1]. A small drop of blood is placed on one coverslip and the second coverslip is placed on top at a 45° angle to the first, making an eight-pointed star when viewed from above. The two coverslips are slid past each other before the blood has fully spread and the resultant smears are air-dried.

Birds

Depending on the size of a bird, one or two people may be required to safely draw blood. If assistance is available, the bird is restrained by one person while the other performs a physical examination or phlebotomy. The bird is restrained around the neck with the thumb under the mandible of the beak and forefinger around the neck. The feet then are held and stretched outwards with the other hand to prevent movement. A towel can be wrapped loosely around the bird to restrict wing movement and may be held with the same hand that holds the head. Care must be taken to ensure that keel movements are not restricted or suffocation may result. If no assistance is available, the bird's body is restrained using a towel. A towel clamp or hemostat can be used to hold the towel securely around the neck [5]. During phlebotomy, the towel is moved to the base of the neck to allow access to the jugular vein (Fig. 1). The bird then is stretched to allow safe access to the jugular vein, while limiting trauma and hematoma formation [5].

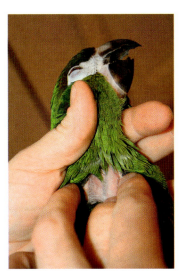

Fig. 1. Two-handed restraint of a Hahn's macaw (*Ara nobilis*) in preparation for drawing blood from the right jugular (j).

Several sites for phlebotomy are available in birds and vary slightly depending on the species. In psittacines, blood typically is obtained from the right jugular vein. Visualization of the jugular is aided by a featherless tract or apteria that lies over the vessel, which also is present in many passerines [5–7]. The left jugular vein is smaller than the right but can be used in medium- to large-sized birds [5,6,8]. Columbiformes do not have a distinct jugular vein in the cervical area, having instead a venous plexus, (*plexus venosus intracutaneous collaris*), which is used for body temperature regulation and behavioral display [6]. Other birds, such as ratites and Anseriformes, lack apteria, making visualization of the jugular vein more difficult [6]. In these birds, the jugular vein may be seen as a swelling in the neck when digital pressure is applied just above the collarbone.

When the jugular vein is not accessible, other sites, such as the basilic and medial metatarsal vein, can be used. The basilic vein is found on the medial aspect of the elbow and is best visualized with a bird in dorsal recumbency and the wing extended (Fig. 2). This vessel is accessible only in medium- to large-sized birds using an insulin syringe or a 25- to 26-gauge needle. This vessel is exceptionally prone to hematoma formation and must be occluded for several minutes to achieve adequate hemostasis [5,6,8].

In larger-sized birds, blood also may be taken with an insulin syringe or 25- to 27-gauge needle on a tuberculin syringe from that medial metatarsal vein, which runs along the medial aspect of the hock [5,6]. Although this site is resistant to hematoma formation, the vessel is prone to bleeding after phlebotomy and may require pressure for 5 to 10 minutes to ensure hemostasis [5,8].

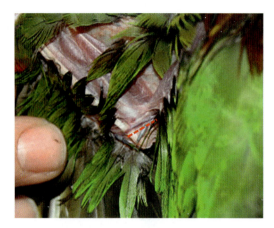

Fig. 2. The right basilic vein can be seen running parallel to the dotted red line in this Hahn's macaw (*Ara nobilis*).

With very small birds, such as budgerigars, canaries, and finches, it may be difficult to access the jugular vein with the aid of an assistant. One person alone can restrain and draw blood. In this technique, the head of a bird is restrained between the forefinger and middle finger while the thumb occludes the jugular vessel at the base of the neck (Fig. 3) [5]. A phlebotomist then draws blood with the dominant hand. After the blood sample has been collected, the syringe is handed to an assistant to prepare samples while the phlebotomist holds off the jugular vein, minimizing hematoma formation.

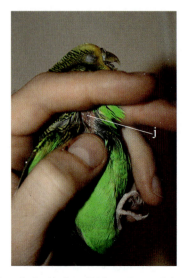

Fig. 3. One-handed restraint of a budgerigar (*Melopsitticus undulatus*) in preparation for drawing blood from the right jugular (j).

In birds weighing less than 60 g, such as budgerigars and lovebirds, an insulin syringe is used to collect blood samples. The authors use insulin syringes whose needle is removable with a hemostat (0.5 mL, 29-gauge needle, reorder #329466, Becton-Dickinson, Franklin Lakes, New Jersey). The needle is removed before depositing the blood into the microtainer to minimize hemolysis. A tuberculin syringe with a 25- to 26-gauge needle is used for slightly larger birds, such as cockatiels and small conures. A 3-mL syringe with a 25-gauge needle is used for larger birds (eg, chickens, ducks, cockatoos, macaws, and Amazon parrots).

Birds have a higher tolerance for blood loss than mammals [9,10]. In general, 1% of a bird's body weight (eg, 1.0 mL from a 100 g bird) may be drawn safely provided it has not recently lost blood or is anemic. Additional blood lost in the formation of a hematoma may be fatal in small birds [5,6]. In the authors' practices, 0.5% of the total body weight generally is drawn, when possible. If the bird's mucous membranes appear pale or if there is a recent history of blood loss, a packed cell volume is measured before phlebotomy using an insulin syringe from the left jugular vein, basilic vein, or medial metatarsal vein. If blood loss from a hematoma is significant, supportive care should be instituted. The bird should be placed in an 85°F incubator and the volume may be replaced with subcutaneous fluids in non-critical cases. More critical cases may require intravenous or intraosseous administration of fluids.

In birds, hematoma formation is a common problem after phlebotomy. The subcutaneous space around the jugular and the basilic is easily distensible and allows for a significant amount of blood loss into this space. In rare cases, this blood loss may be life threatening [5,6].

Snakes

Restraint of snakes for phlebotomy is consistent for all sizes but may be challenging to execute in larger specimens. First, a snake is grasped behind the head to control its movements and prevent bites from aggressive species (eg, blood pythons [Python curtis]). The body of the snake then is held with the other hand. Larger snakes require additional assistants or sedation to hold the body still for phlebotomy. Cardiocentesis is one of the most common methods of phlebotomy in snakes and appears safe [8,11,12]. The snake is positioned in dorsal recumbency and the heart is visualized by observing the cardiac impulse on the ventral surface. The heart then is stabilized between the finger and thumb and the needle introduced underneath a ventral scale approximately one to two scales caudal to where the heart is visualized. The needle is advanced at a 45° angle cranially through skin and into the apex of the ventricle (Fig. 4) [8,11]. Care should be taken not to exert too much negative pressure on the syringe or the ventricles may collapse with possible fatal consequences [12].

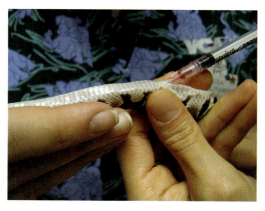

Fig. 4. Cardiocentesis in a ball python (*Python regius*). The head is to the left and the heart is stabilized between the thumb and forefinger.

In snakes weighing more than 300 g, blood is drawn using a 22-gauge needle and a 1- to 3-mL syringe and in snakes weighing less than 300 g, a 25-gauge needle and a 1-mL syringe. A 25-gauge needle is safer for smaller patients but hemolysis is a common complication and artifactually may elevate the potassium [13].

Another site for phlebotomy is the ventral coccygeal vein, located caudal to the vent. When sampling from this site, care should be taken to avoid the paired hemipenes of males, which extend 14 to 16 subcaudal scales caudal to the vent, and the paired musk glands of females, which extend up to six subcaudal scales caudal to the vent [11]. The coccygeal vein can be accessed by placing the needle on the ventral midline and angling between 45° and 60° to the plane of the subcaudal scales. The needle then is inserted and advanced craniodorsally until the needle touches the vertebra. The needle is withdrawn slowly while applying a slight amount of negative pressure. The vessel may be surprisingly superficial when compared with the caudal tail vein in lizards [12]. It is accessed most easily in larger snakes, and lymphatic contamination is possible. Snakes weighing less than 250 g require a 27-gauge, 5/8-inch needle on a 1- to 2-mL syringe, and larger snakes require a 25-gauge needle [11,12].

The palatine-pterygoid vein is another vein described in some texts as a site for phlebotomy. Although it is easily visualized on the dorsal aspect of the oral cavity, it is not acceptable as a site for phlebotomy. It is difficult to access and prone to hematoma formation that occasionally causes anorexia [11,12,14].

Chelonians

There are several veins that may be accessed for phlebotomy in chelonians. These include the jugular, the subcarapacial, and the dorsal tail (coccygeal) vein. Other sites are described, (brachial and femoral veins and plexuses, orbital sinuses, and toenail clips) but are considered of little clinical value because of inadequate sample size or contamination [11,15].

In chelonians, the jugular vein is located running along the neck at the level of the tympanic membrane [8,12]. This location is considerably more dorsal than in mammals (Fig. 5). With the head extended, the jugular vein is held off with a finger or cotton-tipped applicator while a second person draws the blood. The vein may be better visualized by turning the head slightly away from the side of the neck to be sampled. The skin is aseptically prepared with alcohol. The needle is placed just caudal to the tympanum and directed caudally. Digital pressure should be applied to the site after phlebotomy to prevent hematoma formation. The jugular vein is ideal because larger volumes may be collected from this site and the risk of contamination with lymph is minimal; however, it may be difficult to extract and hold the head in most chelonians [11,12,15].

The dorsal tail (coccygeal) vein is accessed by extending the tail and inserting a 25-g needle on the dorsal midline at an angle of 45° to 90° to the plane of the skin and advanced cranially while exerting slight negative pressure on the needle. If the vertebra is encountered, the needle is withdrawn slightly and redirected cranially or caudally. The site is easily accessible but only small blood volumes can be collected and there is a significant risk for lymph contamination [7,11,12,15].

In an uncooperative chelonian whose head and tail are not accessible, the subcarapacial vein may be the easiest site to access. This site is formed by the communication of the cranial-most intercostals vessels and the caudal cervical anastomosis of the left and right jugular veins [11,15]. A 22- to 25-gauge needle is inserted at midline slightly caudal to the area of skin insertion on the ventral aspect of the cranial rim of the carapace (Fig. 6). The needle is advanced caudodorsally with a slight negative pressure. If the vertebrae

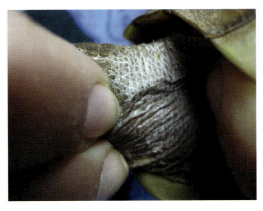

Fig. 5. The jugular vein in a red-eared slider (*Trachemys scripta*). The head is facing to the left.

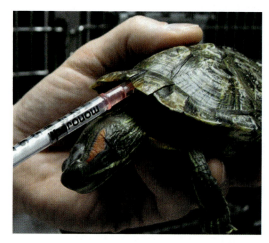

Fig. 6. Phlebotomy in a red-eared slider (*Trachemys scripta*) from the subcarapatial vein.

are encountered, the needle is withdrawn slightly and redirected cranially or caudally. Lymph contamination also is possible at this site [11,15].

Lizards

In lizards, restraint is an important consideration for successful phlebotomy. In many cases, the firmer the grip, the more a lizard struggles [11,16]. Gloves or a towel may be used to protect handlers from sharp nails or bites. Larger lizards, such as iguanas, are restrained on the examination table in a crossed-hands hold. In this method a restrainer crosses hands over the body of an animal and holds the back of the head with one hand and the tail or pelvis with the other. Care must be taken to prevent loss of the tail in those species that are capable of tail autotomy, a defensive adaptation that allows the tail to fracture and detach from the body when grabbed by a predator or restrainer. Some lizards may be relaxed by gently stroking the pineal gland located on the top of the head or by securing cotton balls over their eyes with self adhesive tape, which induces a vasovagal response [11,16]. Smaller lizards may be restrained more easily by using a towel or anesthetized with sevoflurane or isoflurane [16].

The caudal tail vein is the most clinically useful site for phlebotomy in lizards [7,11,12,16,17]. This vessel may be approached from the ventral or lateral aspect of the tail, anywhere from 20% to 80% down its length. If approaching from the ventrum, the needle is positioned along the ventral midline perpendicular to the skin. The needle then is advanced while applying a slight negative pressure. If coccygeal vertebrae are encountered, the needle is withdrawn slightly. If the vein is approached laterally, the lateral processes of the coccygeal vertebrae are palpated and the needle inserted through the skin just ventral to these processes (Fig. 7). Lymphatic contamination may be more likely with the lateral approach [11].

Frogs and salamanders

When restraining amphibians, risks to patients and to handlers must be considered. Defensive secretions of some species may either pose a zoonotic risk or may be poisonous (eg, Cuban tree frogs [*Osteopilus septentrionalis*] and several toads of the *Bufo* genus) [18]. Gloves also prevent calluses and fingerprint ridges from causing abrasion to the sensitive skin of amphibians. To minimize this risk, all gloves are rinsed with distilled water to remove any dust or talc powder before handling and to provide a smooth surface to move against. The gloves also may be covered with a thin coating of a water-soluble nontoxic gel, although this makes them slippery. After use, the gloves should be turned inside out and disposed of in hazardous waste containers [18].

A patient also can be examined by suspending it in a transparent bucket, filled with toxin-free water or water from the patient's enclosure. The bucket should have high walls to prevent escapes in jumping species. Toxin-free water, or water from the patient's enclosure, should be available to moisten patients during an examination in those patients where water from their enclosure is not available [18].

Chemical restraint may be safer and more effective for small amphibians. Isoflurane can be applied topically in a gel form, where 3 mL of isoflurane is mixed with 1.5 mL of water and 3.5 mL of a water-soluble gel (K-Y Jelly, Johnson and Johnson, New Brunswick, New Jersey). This gel is applied topically to the amphibian at a dose of 0.025 mL/g for the aquatic African clawed frog (*Xenopus laevis*) or 0.035 mL/g for the terrestrial *Bufo* species [18,19].

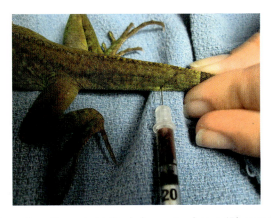

Fig. 7. Phlebotomy from the ventral tail vein in a water dragon (*Physignathus cocincinus*).

Other anesthetic agents are described, the most common being tricaine methanesulfonate (FINQUEL or MS-222, Argent Chemical Laboratories, Redmond, Washington). Tricaine has been used extensively in fish and amphibian medicine, and its properties are well studied. This compound is acidic and should be mixed in a sodium phosphate–buffered solution (Na_2HPO_4, Sigma Scientific, St. Louis, Missouri) to balance the pH. Tricane offers a good plane of anesthesia for most procedures while causing little or no bradycardia, except at deep planes of anesthesia. To prepare a tricaine solution of 0.1% (1 g/L) concentration, 2 L of distilled water, 34 to 50 mL of a 0.5-mol Na_2HPO_4 buffering solution, and 2 g of powdered tricaine methanesulfonate are mixed immediately before use [18]. Induction of adult amphibians usually is achieved within 30 minutes of placing a patient into the 0.1% tricaine solution. After the appropriate anesthetic plane is achieved (generally within 30 minutes), the amphibian is moved from the tricaine solution to water free of tricaine. This often gives enough anesthesia for most diagnostic or surgical procedures. If a patient starts to recover prematurely, it may be placed back into a diluted tricaine solution (0.03%–0.05%) until the appropriate anesthetic plane is achieved [18].

Several sites for phlebotomy exist in amphibians. These include the lingual venous plexus, the midline abdominal vein, the ventral caudal (tail) vein, and the heart [4]. The lingual venus plexus lies immediately under the tongue of many frogs and is reported to work well even in frogs as small as 25 g. The mouth is opened carefully using a rubber spatula, credit card, or mini–cotton-tipped applicator, avoiding fracture of their thin mandibular bones. The tongue then is drawn forward using a cotton-tipped applicator. The venous plexus then can be visualized on the underside of the tongue and buccal floor as a purple-to-red network of veins. The plexus is lacerated with a 25- to 26-gauge needle, and blood is collected in a heparized microhematocrit tube as it oozes out. Releasing the tongue often is adequate to achieve hemostasis. Contamination from oral secretions may occur but can be minimized by swabbing the site with a dry cotton-tipped applicator before venipuncture [4].

The midline ventral abdominal vein is large and runs subcutaneously over the linea alba. A 26- to 27-gauge needle with a 0.5- to 1-mL syringe is inserted craniodorsally into the vein at a level midway between the caudal edge of the sternum and the cranial edge of the pelvis in many frogs and salamanders [4].

The tail vein in salamanders is accessed as described for lizards, using caution to avoid tail autotomy. A 27-gauge needle should be used in animals weighing less than 80 g, and a 25- to 26-gauge needle may be used in larger patients [4].

Cardiocentesis works well in many species and is not a terminal procedure. If an animal is difficult to restrain, it should be anesthetized to minimize risk for damage to the heart and pericardium. While in dorsal recumbency, the cardiac pulse is identified and the apex of the heart is penetrated using a 25-, 26-, or 27-gauge needle and syringe. Slight negative pressure is applied to the syringe as it is advanced until a flash of blood is seen in the hub. The negative pressure on the syringe then is released. A gentle cycle of negative pressure and release helps draw the blood into the syringe with each heartbeat. Contamination with clear to cloudy yellow pericardial fluid can occur, and this pericardial fluid may be saved for cytology or culture, but to get a blood sample, a new needle and syringe should be used for a second attempt. Additional attempts at cardiocentesis increase the risk for damage to the heart and pericardium [4].

Fish

Restraint in fish must be performed carefully. Every effort must be made to avoid tearing the fins, removing scales, and damaging the outermost surface of the skin, composed of mucous and cell debris, called the cuticle [20–23]. The initial examination is performed by visualizing a patient in its environment, where observations are made on a fish's position in the water column, appetite, behavior (huddled near aerator or mouthing at the surface), swimming ability, fin movements, and any gross lesions [20,23]. Scooping a fish from its enclosure into a smaller clear plastic bag or clear plastic container can facilitate some of these observations. After this examination, it may be necessary to remove a fish from the water for a closer examination and for sample collection. Some placid fish may be held out of the water for up to a minute, but many require sedation. When possible, it is best to examine a fish while held over water in case the fish should jump or slips from a handler's grasp [23]. The fish is restrained by grasping by the caudal peduncle (base of the tail) and supported from underneath by the other hand. Care needs to be taken for those fish that possess hard spines to avoid injury [20,23]. Artificial chamois cloth is minimally abrasive and can be used in transporting a fish from one enclosure to another [20].

Sedation in fish also is achieved with tricaine but at a lower concentration than that used for amphibians. Two protocols for preparing the tricaine for use in fishes are described. In the first, tricaine may be added to the fish's water at 50 to 90 mg/L along with an equal volume of sodium bicarbonate to buffer the solution (50 to 90 mg/L) [20]. The second protocol is convenient if larger numbers of procedures are going to be performed. A stock solution of 1% (10 g/L) tricaine is created by adding 20 g of tricaine to 2 L of sodium phosphate buffered water. The stock solution can be stored in a dark bottle and refrigerated for up to 3 months [22]. Ideally, water from which the fish originated should be used, at the same temperature, provided it is clean and free of toxins or waste products [20,22]. This stock solution is more concentrated than that described for amphibians and allows a fish's own water to be used with much less dilution by the tricaine solution. Induction of a fish is achieved at 50- to 200-mg/L tricaine and the fish is maintained at 50 to 100 mg/L [20,21]. During the procedure the water must be well aerated and patients monitored for respiration by observing opercular (gill-covering) movement. For recovery or to achieve a lighter plane of sedation, fish should be removed to water free of tricaine. The fish may be released from restraint when it is able to swim on its own [21].

The most common site for phlebotomy in fish is the caudal vein (Fig. 8). It may be approached laterally or from the ventral midline similar to the manner described in the caudal tail vein of lizards. If the lateral approach is used, the needle is inserted at a point on or just below the lateral line. Syringes that have been rinsed with heparin should be used because fish blood tends to coagulate quickly [21,24].

Ferrets

There are several veins available for phlebotomy in ferrets. Larger volumes may be obtained from the jugular vein or the cranial vena cava and smaller volumes may be obtained from the cephalic and saphenous veins. The authors' vessel of choice is the cranial vena cava. Ferrets have a relatively long thorax, and the heart is located more distal to the site of phlebotomy minimizing the risk for cardiocentesis from this site [25]. In this technique, a ferret is scruffed and held in dorsal recumbancy with a restrainer's hand and the head of the ferret held off the end of the table. The forepaws then are grasped and drawn caudally, keeping two fingers between the forepaws so the legs are not rotated medially [8]. A second person restrains the ferret around the waist just cranial to the pelvis. Restraint of the back feet should be avoided, as this seems to annoy ferrets. The ferret is stretched and laid as flat as possible to minimize movement. Phlebotomy is performed using a 25-gauge needle on a 3-mL syringe. The notch between the first rib and the manubrium of the sternum is identified by resting a finger on the tip of the sternum, then allowing it to fall to laterally into the divot just cranial to the first rib. The needle is held at a 45°angle to the surface of the table and is directed toward the contralateral hip (Fig. 9). Negative pressure is applied to the syringe as it is advanced. Needle advancement is

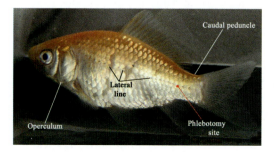

Fig. 8. Photo of a goldfish (*Carassius auratus*), highlighting landmarks for restraint (the caudal peduncle) and for phlebotomy (red dot) on or just ventral to the lateral line.

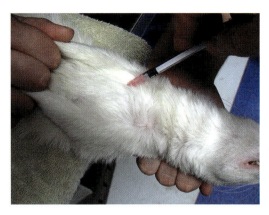

Fig. 9. Phlebotomy of a ferret (*Mustela putorius furo*) from the cranial vena cava. Note how the forearms are restrained with two fingers between them so that they will be spaced farther apart to allow better access to the phlebotomy site. The head (facing to the right) is restrained off to table to allow the ferret's head and neck and body to be in a straight line.

stopped when blood appears in the syringe. If a third person is not available, the ferret is wrapped in a towel up to its axillae allowing a handler to restrain the head and forepaws (described previously) [25].

Care should be taken when drawing blood from the cranial vena cava because serious hemorrhage could occur if a ferret struggles [8,26]. The authors sometimes offer an oil-based liquid treat (eg, Linatone, Church & Dwight, Princeton, New Jersey), which often distracts a ferret long enough to perform the procedure without resistance. Sugar-containing treats (eg, Nutrical, Evsco Pharmaceuticals, division of Vétoquinol, Buena, New Jersey) should be avoided as these elevate the blood glucose values quickly. Ferrets also can be placed under general anesthesia using sevoflurane or isoflurane if they cannot be restrained safely [8,26].

To access the jugular vein, ferrets are restrained in a manner similar to that used in cats. The front legs are extended down over the edge of a table and the neck extended upwards. Visibility of the vein can be enhanced by shaving the neck. The vein in ferrets is located somewhat more laterally than it is in cats. Depending on the size of the ferret, a 22- to 25-gauge needle may be used [26].

The lateral saphenous and cephalic veins may be useful for sampling small volumes of blood but should be avoided if intravenous catheterization is required for patient stabilization. A 27- to 29-gauge needle on an insulin syringe is recommended at this site to help prevent collapse of the vein [26].

Rabbits

Restraint in rabbits must be performed carefully. A rabbit's skeleton comprises 8% of its body weight, whereas a cat's is 13% [8,27]. Rabbit muscles are strong, placing them at increased risk for fractures of the long bones and spine. For this reason it is important to support a rabbit's back during restraint and transport. Two methods of restraint are used to move rabbits over short distances, as from the carrier to the examination table. The first places a rabbit in an upright position with the rabbit's back against the handler's chest, the back legs supported with one hand, and the rabbit's chest supported with the other hand (Fig. 10A). With the second type of restraint, a rabbit is placed in sternal recumbence on one arm with the head held gently against the body with the same elbow. The other hand is placed gently but squarely on the neck of the rabbit (see Fig. 10B) [27].

Blood may be drawn from several sites on the rabbit. The jugular vein is a convenient site in some rabbits because it allows for a larger volume of blood (>0.5 mL) to be drawn quickly. Rabbit are restrained in a similar way to cats, with the neck extended upwards and the feet drawn straight

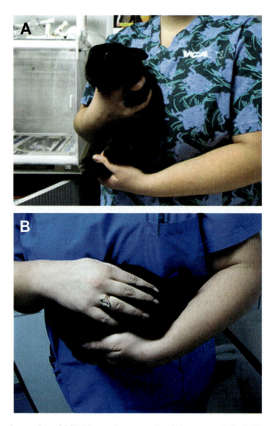

Fig. 10. (*A*) The domestic rabbit (*Oryctolagus cuniculi*) is supported at three points: its chest with one hand, its back against the handler's chest, and its pelvis with the other hand. This prevents the rabbit from injuring itself by trying to kick. (*B*) The football hold, with the head of the rabbit tucked into the handler's left elbow, the body supported with the left hand and arm, and the right hand lightly but surely restraining the head and neck.

down over the edge of the table. Care must be taken not to overextend the head because this may cause difficulty breathing. The jugular vein may be inaccessible in female rabbits and some obese male rabbits when a substantial dewlap is present [8,27].

The lateral saphenous vein can be accessed easily and with minimal stress to the rabbit. In this technique, a rabbit is restrained at the edge of the table with its head between a restrainer's elbow and body (Fig. 11A). The leg is extended over the edge of the table and held at the crux of the stifle to occlude venous return. The vein is superficial, easily visualized, and often entered immediately as the needle pierces the skin (see Fig. 11B). It is prone to hematoma formation, so it should be held off well after phlebotomy [8,27].

The marginal ear vein also is easily accessible but is very small and can collapse. Small samples can be obtained, however, with minimal restraint and stress to the rabbit. Thrombosis and consequential sloughing of a small portion of the pinna is a rare complication [7,27].

Guinea pigs

Restraint for physical examination in guinea pigs is easy. Many guinea pigs are restrained adequately simply by grasping them securely around the shoulders and thorax or by wrapping in a towel [25].

Blood collection in guinea pigs is more challenging. The most readily accessible vessels for phlebotomy are the lateral saphenous and cephalic veins.

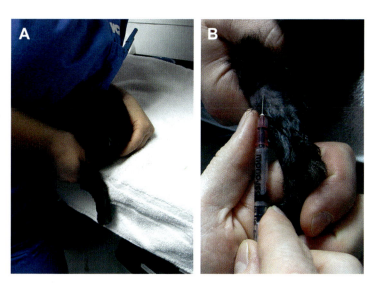

Fig. 11. (*A*) Restraint of the domestic rabbit (*Oryctolagus cuniculi*) in preparation for drawing blood from the lateral saphenous vein. (*B*) Phlebotomy from the lateral saphenous vein of the domestic rabbit.

These are small vessels, however, allowing for only minimal amounts of blood collection and are sites for intravenous catheter placement [28]. Shaving the fur from these areas and wetting the skin with alcohol enhances the visibility of the veins.

The jugular vein is much larger and can be used to collect blood samples, but the restraint necessary to access the vein is stressful [25]. In addition, the necks are short, making location of the jugular a more difficult. Restraint is achieved by extending the head and neck up with the forelegs extended down over the edge of the table. Shaving the neck of guinea pigs aids in visualizing the vein. Patients must be observed closely for signs of dyspnea, stress or collapse. If any of these signs are observed, the procedure must be aborted immediately [25,28].

The cranial vena cava is another vessel available for phlebotomy. Anesthesia is required for proper restraint, however. Sevoflurane or isoflurane typically is used because of rapid induction and recovery times. For phlebotomy of the vena cava, the needle is directed into the thoracic inlet at approximately 30° off of midline and aimed toward the opposite hind leg. In guinea pigs, the heart is close to the site of phlebotomy, so there is an increased risk for hemorrhage into the thoracic cavity or pericardium [28]; however, inadvertent cardiac puncture rarely is associated with severe complications or death [25]. To minimize the risk, small, short needles (1/2 to 5/8 inch) can be used and may be too short to reach the heart [25].

Small rodents

Several sites are used in research animals (rats, mice, hamsters, and gerbils) that are not commonly used in clinical practice. The retro-orbital venous sinus may be used to collect significant volumes of blood, up to 0.5 mL in rats, using a microhematocrit tube. In mice and gerbils, the conjunctiva is penetrated at the medial canthus of the eye, whereas in hamsters and rats the conjunctiva is penetrated midway along the superior border or the eye. Pressure is applied over the eye after the tube is removed to prevent retrobulbar hemorrhage [29,30]. Retro-orbital phlebotomy is controversial in clinical practice because of the potential risk for damage to the eye and surrounding tissues. A skilled phlebotomist can perform the technique such that there are no scars histologically detectable 4 weeks after phlebotomy [31]. When performed by an experienced clinician, the stress to the rodent seems minimal [32]. Opportunities to become proficient at this procedure in a clinical setting are rare, so this remains predominantly a research tool.

In clinical practice, the lateral tail veins and ventral caudal tail artery are used in rats and mice. Vasodilation can be used to help visualize the veins by placing patients in a warm (104°F) incubator for 5 to 10 minutes or placing the tail in a warm water bath. When accessing the tail artery, restraint is achieved with inhalant anesthesia. Before sampling, the plunger of the syringe should be removed. The ventral artery fills a syringe without negative pressure resulting from higher blood pressure [29]. After obtaining a sample, pressure must be applied to the venipuncture site for a longer period of time to ensure adequate hemostasis. When accessing the lateral tail veins, inhalant anesthesia or a modified 50-mL syringe case (the plastic container in which the syringe is stored before use to maintain sterility) with breathing holes punched into the closed end should be used for restraint. A rubber band may be used as a tourniquette to help access the deeper vein [33].

A technique for drawing blood from the lateral saphenous vein also has been described [33,34]. This minimally invasive technique does not require anesthesia and can be performed by a single individual. The hair is clipped from the lateral surface of the hind limb and a patient restrained using a modified 50-mL syringe case or inhalant anesthesia. The hind leg then is extended and the vein occluded by grasping the skin above the stifle. The vein is exposed by wetting the surface with silicon grease or alcohol. Silicon grease is advantageous because it reduces the risk for clotting as the blood contacts the skin. The vessel then is punctured using a 25-gauge needle held at 90° to the skin. A drop of blood appears on the skin and may be collected into hematocrit tubes. When finished, the leg may be released and this typically achieves hemostasis. The site can be accessed multiple times by simply wiping off the scab that forms [33,34].

Hedgehogs

The African hedgehog (*Atelerix albiventris*) and European hedgehog (*Erinaceus europaeus*) are increasingly popular as pets. Restraint for physical examination and phlebotomy may be challenging because they are prone to curling up in a ball and raising their spines. Methods for encouraging a hedgehog to unfurl are described elsewhere in this issue and include placing a curledup hedgehog in a standing position and rocking it up and down in a see-saw fashion, stroking the spines on the rump, and placing it in a small amount of standing water in a clear bucket [35,36]. None of these methods, however, has proved sufficient for phlebotomy. To achieve proper restraint and positioning, anesthesia with sevoflurane or isoflurane is recommended. With a hedgehog in a curled position, a large dog anesthesia mask may be placed over the hedgehog to use as an induction chamber. As a hedgehog becomes anesthetized and uncurled, a smaller mask is placed over the face to maintain the hedgehog at an appropriate level of anesthesia. Hypersalivation can occur with isoflurane as a result of irritation to the mucus membranes. If available, sevoflurane may be used or administration of atropine may be indicated [36,37].

The most accessible veins for phlebotomy are the jugular vein and the cranial vena cava. Because of the propensity for obesity in hedgehogs, the jugular vein may be difficult to visualize. It is located midway between the point of the shoulder and the ramus of the mandible and can be accessed using a 22- to 25-gauge needle on a 1- to 3-mL syringe [36,37]. The cranial vena cava is sampled by inserting a 25-gauge needle at the thoracic inlet, pointing toward the opposite hind leg, 30° off midline. Sampling from the vena cava requires care to prevent laceration of the vessel or damage to other structures of the thoracic inlet and heart [36,37].

Smaller volumes of blood may be obtained from peripheral veins, such as the cephalic, lateral saphenous, and femoral veins; however, the veins tend to collapse easily [36,37].

Sugar gliders

Restraint and phlebotomy of sugar gliders can be challenging. They are more active in the evening than in the morning, so if possible, appointments should be scheduled in the morning hours. Restraint for a physical examination is described as grasping the base of the tail and cupping the body in a hand or towel [38]. For phlebotomy, the authors use sevoflurane or isoflurane anesthesia, delivered by mask.

As with many other small mammals, the two most commonly used sites for blood collection are the jugular vein and the cranial vena cava [37,38]. A large volume of blood may be obtained from either of these sites, up to 1 mL in an adult male sugar glider. The jugular vein is found be directing the needle midway between the point of the shoulder and the ramus of the mandible. The cranial vena cava is accessed by inserting a needle through the skin at the thoracic inlet. The needle should be directed toward the opposite back leg at an approximately 30° angle off midline. As with hedgehogs and guinea pigs, the risks of using the cranial vena cava include accidental cardiocentesis and damage to the vein and other thoracic structures.

Giant spiders (tarantulas)

The body of a giant spider is divided into two sections, the prosoma (fused head and thorax segments), and the opisthosoma or abdomen [39,40]. The eight legs extend off of the prosoma. Giant spiders are susceptible to injury by falls, so care must be taken during restraint. Initial examination should be performed by placing a spider in a clear plastic or glass container, allowing the spider to be viewed from all angles. Restraint also can be achieved by gently grasping the prosoma of a spider with long rubber-tipped tongs. This causes the spider to become nearly immobile with the legs in extension, a reflex believed to lessen its rate of descent during a fall [40]. Handlers should avoid holding the spider too close the face because some species are capable of flicking painful urticating hairs. In addition, many giant spiders are capable of inflicting a painful bite. Anesthesia with isoflurane or sevoflurane may be required for a more thorough physical examination and for drawing hemolymph.

Hemolymph can be sampled in giant spiders. It is a clear to slightly blue fluid that uses hemocyanin, an oxygen-carrying pigment, to store and transport oxygen. Samples may be collected for analysis or for transfusion into another hypovolemic giant spider [39–41]. The amount of hemolymph that can be reasonably collected from a healthy giant spider is 0.6% to 0.7% of its body weight (0.09 mL to 0.1 mL in a 15 g spider) [41].

There are two locations for obtaining hemolymph. The first and most often used is from the heart, located mid-dorsally within the opisthosoma. Spiders are anesthetized with isoflurane or sevoflurane, and a syringe with a 27- to 29-gauge needle is inserted along the dorsal midline of the opisthosoma at its highest point, approximately 45° to the surface of the cuticle (Fig. 12). The advantage to this site is that a large volume of hemolymph may be collected quickly. The disadvantage is that movement by a spider or phlebotomist may result in laceration of the heart and potentially life-threatening exsanguination [39,40].

A second location for very small volumes (possibly enough for a hemolymph smear) is the ventral joint membrane of one of the spider's limbs. Spiders are immobilized in dorsal recumbency with a plastic ruler or similar object. The ventral joint membrane is then penetrated with a 29-g insulin syringe. A significant risk of this procedure is loss of the limb by autotomy [39]. Leg autotomy is an adaptation for escape from predators by voluntarily dropping a limb that is grasped or stung, two events that may be mimicked by hemolymph sampling. This risk is significant enough that some clinicians do not recommend using this site [40].

Summary

Blood sampling is an important diagnostic tool and proper restraint is essential for the safety of patients and handlers. Learning the commonly used sites for phlebotomy in nontraditional pet species, the advantages and disadvantages of each site, and how to access them provide more options in obtaining samples. Multiple options are especially valuable in

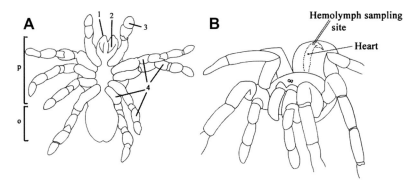

Fig. 12. (*A*) Diagram of the ventral surface of a giant spider (suborder *Mygalomorphae*) showing the cephalothorax or prosoma (p), the abdomen or opisthosoma (o), the chelicera (1), the fangs (2), the pedipalps (3), and the walking legs (4). (*B*) Diagram showing the location of the heart within the opisthosoma and the site for hemolymph sampling.

exotic patients whose small size and unique anatomy make these veins difficult to see and puncture.

Acknowledgments

The author wishes to acknowledge Jessica Honeywell for her excellent technical assistance in restraint and phlebotomy. Her help was greatly appreciated.

References

[1] Fudge AM. Avian blood sampling and artifact considerations. In: Fudge AM, editor. Laboratory medicine avian and exotic pets. St. Louis (MO): Saunders Publishing; 2000. p. 1–8.

[2] Campbell TW. Avian hematology. In: Campbell TW, editor. Avian hematology and cytology. 2nd edition. Ames IA: Iowa State University Press; 1995. p. 3–19.

[3] Campbell TW. Clinical pathology of reptiles. In: Mader DR, editor. Reptile medicine and surgery. 2nd edition. St. Louis (MO): Saunders Publishing; 2006. p. 453–70.

[4] Wright KM. Amphibian hematology. In: Wright KM, Whitaker BR, editors. Amphibian medicine and captive husbandry. Malabar (FL): Krieger Publishing Co; 2001. p. 129–46.

[5] Brown C. Venipuncture in psittacine birds. Lab Anim 2007;36(10):21–2.

[6] Echols S. Collecting diagnostic samples in avian patients. Vet Clin North Am Exot Anim Pract 1999;2(3):621–50.

[7] Sjoberb JG, Odberg E. One perspective on selected blood collection sites in exotic species. Exotic DVM 2003;5(4):27–31.

[8] Briscoe JA, Syring R. Techniques for emergency airway and vascular access in special species. Seminars in Avian and Exotic Pet Medicine 2004;13(3):118–31.

[9] Campbell TW. Hematology. In: Ritchie BW, Harrison GJ, Harrison LR, editors. Avian medicine: principles and application. Lake Worth (FL): Wingers Publishing; 1994. p. 176–98.

[10] Lichtenberger MK, Chavez W, Cray C, et al. Mortality and response to fluid resuscitation after acute blood loss in mallard ducks (Anas platythynnchos). Proceedings of the Annual Conference of the Association of Avian Veterinarians 2003;7–10.

[11] Hernandez-Divers SJ. Diagnostic techniques. In: Mader DR, editor. Reptile medicine and surgery. St. Louis (MO): Saunders Publishing; 2006. p. 490–532.

[12] Redrobe S, MacDonald J. Sample collection and clinical pathology of reptiles. Vet Clin North Am Exot Anim Pract 1999;2(3):709–30.

[13] Wilkinson R. Clinical pathology. In: McArthur S, Wilkinson R, Meyer J, et al, editors. Medicine and surgery of tortoises and turtles. Ames (IA): Blackwell Publishing, Ltd.; 2004. p. 141–86.

[14] Diethelm G. Reptiles. In: Carpenter JW, editor. Exotic animal formulary. 3rd edition. St Louis (MO): Elsevier Inc; 2005. p. 54–131.

[15] Barrows M, McArthur S, Wilkinson R. Diagnosis. In: McArthur S, Wilkinson R, Meyer J, et al, editors. Medicine and surgery of tortoises and turtles. Ames (IA): Blackwell Publishing, Ltd; 2004. p. 109–40.

[16] Barten SL. Lizards. In: Mader DR, editor. Reptile medicine and surgery. 2nd edition. St. Louis (MO): Saunders Publishing; 2006. p. 59–77.

[17] Brown C. Blood sample collection in lizards. Lab Anim 2007;36(8):23–4.

[18] Wright KM. Restraint techniques and euthanasia. In: Wright KM, Whitaker BR, editors. Amphibian medicine and captive husbandry. Malabar (FL): Krieger Publishing Co; 2001. p. 111–28.

[19] Stetter MD, Raphael B, Indiviglio F, et al. Isoflurane anesthesia in amphibians: comparison of five application methods. Proceedings of the American Association of Zoo Veterinarians 1996;255–7.

[20] Weber SE, Innis C. Piscine patients: basic diagnostics. Compendium on Contininuing Education for the Practicing Veterinarian 2007;29(5):276–88.

[21] Johnson D. Practical koi and goldfish medicine. Exotic DVM 2005;6(3):42–8.
[22] Ross LG. Restraint, anaesthesia and euthanasia. In: Wildgoose WH, editor. BSAVA manual of ornamental fish. 2nd edition. Waterwells, Gloucester (UK): British Small Animal Veterinary Association Publishing; 2001. p. 75–83.
[23] Lewbart GA. Clinical examination. In: Wildgoose WH, editor. BSAVA manual of ornamental fish. 2nd edition. Waterwells, Gloucester (UK): British Small Animal Veterinary Association Publishing; 2001. p. 85–9.
[24] Southgate PJ. Laboratory techniques. In: Wildgoose WH, editor. BSAVA manual of ornamental fish. 2nd edition. Waterwells, Gloucester (UK): British Small Animal Veterinary Association Publishing; 2001. p. 91–101.
[25] Lennox AM. Venipuncture in small exotic companion mammals. Clinician's Brief 2007; 5(10):23–6.
[26] Quesenberry KE, Orcutt C. Basic approach to veterinary care. In: Quesenberry KE, Carpenter JW, editors. Ferrets, rabbits, and rodents, clinical medicine and surgery. 2nd edition. St. Louis (MO): Saunders Publishing; 2005. p. 13–24.
[27] Mader DR. Basic approach to veterinary care. In: Quesenberry KE, Carpenter JW, editors. Ferrets, rabbits, and rodents, clinical medicine and surgery. 2nd edition. St. Louis (MO): Saunders Publishing; 2005. p. 147–54.
[28] Quesenberry KE, Donnelly TM, Hillyer EV. Biology, husbandry, and clinical techniques of guinea pigs and chinchillas. In: Quesenberry KE, Carpenter JW, editors. Ferrets, rabbits, and rodents, clinical medicine and surgery. 2nd edition. St. Louis (MO): Saunders Publishing; 2005. p. 232–44.
[29] McClure DE. Clinical pathology and sample collection in the laboratory rodent. Vet Clin North Am Exot Anim Pract 1999;2(3):565–90.
[30] van Herck H, Baumans V, Brandt CJ, et al. Orbital sinus blood sampling in rats as performed by different animal technicians: the influence of technique and expertise. Lab Anim 1998; 32(4):377–86.
[31] van Herck H, Baumans V, van der Craats NR, et al. Histological changes in the orbital region of rats after orbital puncture. Lab Anim 1992;26(1):53–8.
[32] van Herck H, Baumans V, de Boer SF, et al. Endocrine stress response in rats subjected to singular orbital puncture while under diethyl-ether anaesthesia. Lab Anim 1991;25:325–9.
[33] Bihun C, Bauck L. Basic anatomy, physiology, husbandry, and clinical techniques. In: Quesenberry KE, Carpenter JW, editors. Ferrets, rabbits and rodents, clinical medicine and surgery. 2nd edition. St.Louis (MO): Saunders Publishing; 2005. p. 286–98.
[34] Hem A, Smith AJ, Solberg P. Saphenous vein puncture for blood sampling of the mouse, rat, hamster, gerbil, guinea pig, ferret and mink. Lab Anim 1998;32:364–8.
[35] Johnson-Delaney CA. Hedgehogs. In: Johnson-Delaney CA, editor. Exotic companion medicine handbook for veterinarians. Lake Worth (FL): Zoological Education Network; 2005. p. 1–14.
[36] Ivey E, Carpenter JW. African hedgehogs. In: Quesenberry KE, Carpenter JW, editors. Ferrets, rabbits and rodents, clinical medicine and surgery. 2nd edition. St.Louis (MO): Saunders Publishing; 2005. p. 339–53.
[37] Ness RD. Clinical pathology and sample collection of exotic small mammals. Vet Clin North Am Exot Anim Pract 1999;2(3):591–620.
[38] Ness RD. Sugar gliders. In: Quesenberry KE, Carpenter JW, editors. Ferrets, rabbits and rodents, clinical medicine and surgery. 2nd edition. St.Louis (MO): Saunders Publishing; 2005. p. 330–8.
[39] Pizzi R. Spiders. In: Lewbart GA, editor. Invertebrate medicine. Ames (IA): Blackwell Publishing; 2006. p. 143–68.
[40] Johnson-Delaney CA. Tarantulas. In: Johnson-Delaney CA, editor. Exotic companion medicine handbook for veterinarians. Lake Worth (FL): Zoological Education Network; 2005. p. 1–26.
[41] Visigalli G. Observations from the field: guide to hemolymph transfusion in giant spiders. Exotic DVM 2004;5(6):42–3.

ELSEVIER
SAUNDERS

VETERINARY
CLINICS
Exotic Animal Practice

Vet Clin Exot Anim 11 (2008) 445–462

Hematologic Disorders of Fish

Tonya M. Clauss, DVM, MS[a],*,
Alistair D.M. Dove, PhD[a], Jill E. Arnold, MS, MT[b]

[a]*Veterinary Services and Conservation Medicine, Georgia Aquarium, 225 Baker Street,
Atlanta, GA 30313, USA*
[b]*National Aquarium in Baltimore, Pier 3, 501 East Pratt Street, Baltimore, MD 21202, USA*

Most fish health research and medicine traditionally has focused on aquaculture and food fish species. As society recognizes the need for conserving and protecting its natural resources, public aquarium facilities, commercial ornamental fish producers, collectors, and hobbyists are following the lead of the aquaculture industry by improving fish health practices for popular display fish. The growth of domestic animal medicine as a discipline over the past few decades also has had an impact on fish medicine. Pets, including fish, often are believed members of the family and, as a result, more private practitioners are being consulted about pet fish health. Hematologic data not always have been used in evaluating fish health because of the difficulty of obtaining samples, the challenges involved in evaluating hemograms, and the lack of meaningful reference intervals to aid in interpretation. Hematologic evaluation can be useful in monitoring the health status of fish, as long as interpretation accounts for intrinsic and extrinsic factors that can influence the appearance of cells and the quantitative values obtained. Care must be taken when comparing data as many published reference ranges do not account for differences attributed to factors, such as age, gender, water quality, and season. Even the capture, handling, and anesthetics involved in obtaining blood samples from fish can have profound affects on the hemogram [1].

Hematologic disorders are marked by aberrations in structure or function of the blood cells or the mechanisms of coagulation. Although many other diseases may be reflected by the blood and its constituents, the abnormalities of erythrocytes, leukocytes, thrombocytes, and clotting factors are considered primary blood disorders. Diseases of fish may result in anemia, leukopenia, leukocytosis, thrombocytopenia, and other blood cell abnormalities.

* Corresponding author.
E-mail address: tclauss@georgiaaquarium.org (T.M. Clauss).

1094-9194/08/$ - see front matter © 2008 Elsevier Inc. All rights reserved.
doi:10.1016/j.cvex.2008.03.007 *vetexotic.theclinics.com*

This article summarizes some of the salient features of hematologic analysis in teleosts (bony fishes) and elasmobranchs (sharks and rays) and outlines the ways in which the major types of diseases can present themselves in a fish hemogram. Blood sample collection and handling techniques for both classes of fishes are described in the literature [2–5] and are not discussed further in this review.

Normal erythrocytes

Erythrocytes of teleost fishes have similar appearance and ultrastructure to those of other nonmammalian vertebrates. The cells are oval to elliptic in shape with abundant pale, eosinophilic cytoplasm and centrally positioned oval to elliptic nuclei, which is moderately to deeply basophilic (Fig. 1). Elasmobranch erythrocytes are similar in appearance to those of teleosts but considerably larger (Fig. 2). A small amount of erythropoiesis occurs in the peripheral blood of both classes of fish, so it is common to find a small percentage of immature erythrocytes when examining a hemogram from a normal fish [6,7]. Moderate anisocytosis and polychromasia also is normal in many species of teleosts and elasmobranchs. Immature erythrocytes tend to be more rounded than oval with a blue-tinted cytoplasm and larger, more heterochromatic nucleus, thus a higher nucleus to cytoplasm ratio. Erythrocyte morphology, interspecific variation, and variations noted in response to intrinsic and extrinsic variables are summarized in detail in existing literature [4,5].

Techniques for laboratory evaluation of erythrocytes also are well described [4,5,8,9]. Examining morphology, determining the packed cell volume (PCV), and obtaining total erythrocyte counts and red blood cell indices, such as mean cell volume, mean corpuscular hemoglobin concentration, and mean corpuscular hemoglobin, all can be useful in diagnosing disease. PCV varies within and between species and seems to correlate with the normal activity level of the fish. For example, actively swimming species, such as tuna and other pelagic species, tend to have much higher PCVs than would a sedentary bottom dweller, such as a flatfish. Elasmobranchs have lower concentrations of larger cells and usually have lower PCVs. As with other hematologic parameters, PCV values may vary with age, gender, water quality, photoperiod, diet, and season [10–17]. In the absence of established reference ranges, an accepted PCV range for fish is 20% to 45% [17].

Normal leukocytes

Leukocytes of fishes are variable between species (see Figs. 1 and 2), such that initially it can be hard to identify some cell types. The main leukocytes can be identified using a comparative approach and process of elimination on a typical blood smear processed with a three-step Romanowsky-type

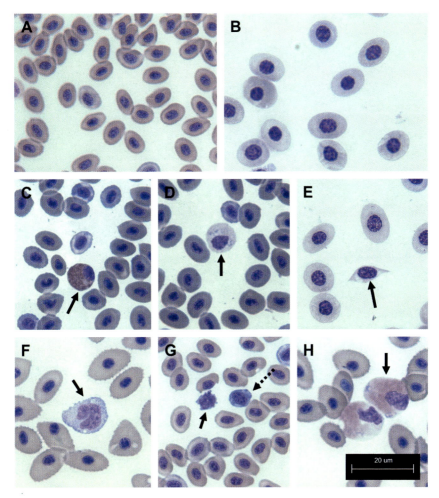

Fig. 1. Normal teleost blood cell morphology. (*A*) Mature erythrocyte morphology of golden trevally, *Gnathanodon speciosus*. (*B*) Mature erythrocyte morphology of ocean sunfish *Mola mola*, showing comparatively larger cells. (*C*) Eosiniophil of a goatfish *Upeneus* sp showing marginal nucleus and large cigar-shaped eosinophilic granules. (*D*) Neutrophil of goatfish showing pale cytoplasm with sparse granulation (some basophily in this case) and eccentric unsegmented nucleus. (*E*) Thrombocyte of ocean sunfish showing spindle shape typical of many teleost thrombocytes. (*F*) Monocyte of the arowana *Osteoglossum bichirrosum* showing typical indented nucleus and abundant vacuolated basophillic cytoplasm. (*G*) Mature lymphocyte (*solid arrow*) and immature erythrocyte (*dashed arrow*) of golden trevally. Note that the immature erythrocyte nucleus is essentially similar to that of mature erythrocytes and that, despite the similar basophilic nature, there is comparatively more cytoplasm in the immature erythrocyte. (*H*) Heterophils of the arowana showing pale basophillic cytoplasm and abundant tiny eosinophillic granules. These cells may fill the same roles as the neutrophils in (*D*) (see text for further discussion).

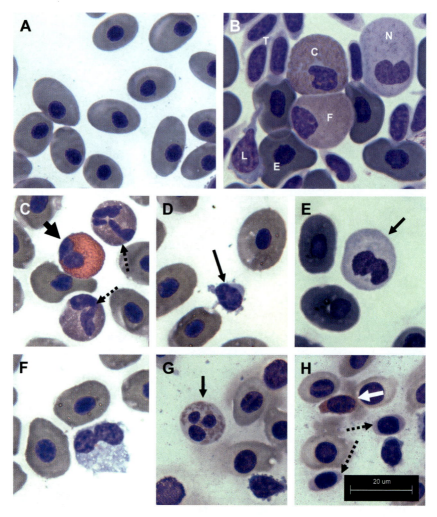

Fig. 2. Normal elasmobranch blood cell morphology. (*A*) Mature erythrocyte morphology of bonnet head shark, *Sphyrna tiburo*, note throughout the plate that erythrocytes are much larger than those of teleosts shown in Fig. 1. (*B*) Buffy coat smear from the whale shark, *Rhinchodon typus,* showing erythrocytes (E), a lymphocyte (L), heterophil (F), eosinophil (C), neutrophil (N) and thromboytes (T). (*C*) Eosinophil or CEG (*solid arrow*) and two heterophils or FEG (*dashed arrows*) in the blood of a southern ray, *Dasyatis americana*. The granules of the CEG have vivid eosinophilic properties and are larger and cigar shaped. (*D*) Lymphocyte (*arrow*) of southern ray showing sparse basophilic cytoplasm, dense nucleus and blebbing of the plasma membrane. (*E*) Neutrophil of spotted wobbegong, *Orectolobus maculatus*. (*F*) Monocyte of the southern ray showing typical indented nucleus and abundant vacuolated basophillic cytoplasm. (*G*) CEG of the carcharhinid black tip shark *Carcharhinus melanopterus*. This cell type has larger granules similar to the eosniophil or CEG of other shark orders, but the tinctorial properties are more similar to the heterophil or FEG found in other orders. The same applies to carcharhinid FEGs, which display vivid eosinophilia, despite their smaller granules. The homologies of these two cell types with the CEG and FEG of other elasmobranch orders have not been established. (*H*) Thrombocytes in the blood of the black tip shark. Both granular (*white arrow*) and agranular (*dashed arrows*) thrombocytes occur in this species.

hematology stain. Evaluation of ultrastructure and thorough review of fish leukoctyes in the literature has alleviated some of the confusion and difficulty associated with hemogram evaluation. Teleost and elasmobranch leukocytes are discussed briefly. In-depth summaries of identification and laboratory evaluation can be found in the literature [2,4,5,8,9,18].

Lymphocytes are the most common and probably most variable leukocyte in most healthy teleosts and elasmobranchs. These are small cells with densely basophilic nuclei and, usually, a very small amount of distinctly blue cytoplasm; the nucleus-to-cytoplasm ratio is high. They sometimes are rounded but often irregular in shape and often with "blebs" or blister-like outpocketings of the outer membrane. Reactive lymphocytes are larger and plasma cells do occur and can appear 2 to 3 times larger than regular lymphocytes [9].

The most common granulocyte of teleosts is the neutrophil. These typically are rounded cells that have nuclei that may or may not be segmented and their cytoplasm varies from extremely pale to gray or slightly blue, depending on the species [19]. The nucleus-cytoplasm ratio is low and cells tend to be similar to or larger than erythrocytes, rarely if ever smaller. Granulation also varies from indistinct to obvious, with the granules themselves appearing anywhere from glassy to slightly eosinophilic or basophilic. Some cell populations with more prominent eosinophilic granules can resemble heterophils of birds and reptiles or the heterophil or fine eosinophilic granulocyte (FEG) of elasmobranchs. Campbell [4] and Campbell and Ellis [5], however, conclude that there are enough functional studies to show that these cells fill the neutrophil role in the teleost leukocyte panoply. Although immature neutrophils occur in the circulating blood of teleosts, they do not resemble the classic band cell of the mammalian leukogram. In typical neutrophils and heterophils, the nucleus may be segmented or nonsegmented in mature cells depending on species and, sometimes, within a species. Neutrophils also are found commonly in elasmobranch species. The nuclei can be lobed or round. The cytoplasm is colorless with no visible granulation [8,9].

True eosinophils are less common in teleosts whereas basophils are rare. The granules of eosinophils tend to be larger and more distinct than those of the neutrophil/heterophil series, round or rod-shaped, and prominently eosinophilic; they are not easily overlooked. Basophils, when they occur, contain granules that stain so darkly as to obscure the nucleus [4]. In contrast, elasmobranchs show abundant eosinophilic cells, generally falling into two morphologic types. Consistent in sharks and rays is a cell that closely resembles the avian heterophils, with elongated, rod-shaped granules that stain a reddish color in Romanowsky-type stains. Nomenclature varies in the literature; this article uses the terminology described by Hine and Wain [20,21] as FEG. The second cell type, termed coarse eosinophilic granulocyte (CEG), is of equal size, but the granules are round and usually less abundant in the cytoplasm. The staining properties vary with species; most shark and ray CEGs stain orange to bright orange whereas the carhcharinid

CEG granules stain pale pink. The nuclei can be lobed or round in the FEG and CEG cells. Basophils rarely, if ever, are present in shark species but commonly found in rays. Elasmobranch leukocyte function warrants further study.

Monocytes of teleosts and elasmobranchs are similar to those of other vertebrates; they probably are the largest cells in any differential, irregular in shape, with an eccentric, large, heterochromatic nucleus (often indented or kidney shaped) and abundant slightly basophilic cytoplasm replete with vacuoles and other membrane-bound organelles.

Abnormalities of erythrocytes and leukocytes

Hematologic abnormalities involving the erythrocytes of fish include polycythemia, anemia, abnormal morphology, and nuclear or cytoplasmic inclusions. Like other vertebrates, fish leukograms are affected by disease, inflammatory processes, stress, nutrition, and physiologic and environmental factors. During disease processes, the leukogram of teleosts can show many of the patterns that are seen in mammals, although Campbell and Ellis [5] stress that the exact functions of piscine granulocytes are not established, so direct comparisons with mammalian processes are somewhat speculative.

Polycythemia and anemia

Fish with a PCV of 45% or greater generally are considered to have a relative polycythemia resulting from dehydration, especially when in conjunction with an elevation in serum osmolality, total protein, sodium, or chloride. Polycythemia also can be observed, however, in sexually mature males, in freshwater fish exposed to hypoxia, in stressed fish resulting from release of catecholamines, during splenic contraction, and with erythrocyte swelling [6,22,23].

Anemias are well documented in fish. PCVs less than 20% in teleosts usually are associated with anemia. Diagnosing anemias in elasmobranchs can be more challenging as some species have a normal PCV of 20% or less (for example, sandbar shark [*Carcharhinus plumbeus*] and the Port Jackson shark [*Heterodontus portusjacksoni*]) [2,9]. The PCV of some sharks varies between blood collection sites and this possibility should be taken into account when diagnosing anemia [24]. There are three primary types of anemia: hemorrhagic (blood loss), hemolytic (erythrocyte destruction), and hypoplastic (poor erythropoiesis). The basic descriptive terminology used for anemias in other animals applies equally to fishes and may refer to cell size (microcytic, normocytic, or macrocytic), hemoglobin concentration (hypochromic or normochromic), cell loss (hemolytic or hemorrhagic), and hemopoietic status (regenerative or nonregenerative). Causes of nonregenerative anemias include inflammatory disease, nutritional disorders, toxins, and renal or splenic disease with disruption or destruction of hematopoietic tissues.

The specific hematologic presentation of a given anemia often provides indications as to the etiology of the disease.

Marked hemorrhage or hemolysis often results in microcytic anemia because regenerating immature erythrocytes make up the majority of cells in peripheral circulation and are smaller in size than mature erythrocytes. Marked polychromasia also may be noted. The presence of immature erythrocytes in circulation does not always signify a regenerative anemia; immature cells may be present in response to environmental stressors, such as hypoxia, toxins, or temperature change [18,25–27]. Hemorrhagic anemia in fish may be associated with trauma, cutaneous ulceration, parasitism (lampreys, leeches, and isopods) [5,28], nutritional deficiencies (vitamin K and B, inositol, and choline) [5,18], and viral or bacterial septicemia (Tables 1 and 2). When severe or chronic blood loss occurs, the net loss of iron may result in iron deficiency anemia. Hemolytic anemia in fish may be associated with hemolysin-producing bacteria (see Table 1), environmental toxins [29–31], viral infection [32], select nutritional deficiencies [33–35], and hemoparasites [3–5,36,37]. Marked regeneration often is noted with hemolytic anemia because the iron is not lost from the body and can be incorporated back into hemoglobin for hematopoiesis. Erythrocytes with pyknotic nuclei, erythroplastids, and erythrocyte fragmentation are associated with conditions that interfere with splenic removal of senescent erythrocytes from peripheral circulation [38]. Table 1 provides an overview of various causes and clinical presentations of anemia in teleosts.

Intrinsic and extrinsic induced variability

Stress factors in fish are as variable as they are with other animals. Extrinsic factors, such as handling, transport, poor water quality, and high population densities, initially may cause a significant stress response in most fish but with chronicity or acclimation the response may diminish. Stress response in fish is similar to that of higher vertebrates with a rapid release of catecholamines followed by the release of corticosteroids. A stress leukogram for most fish is manifested as a leukopenia with a lymphopenia and a relative granulocytosis. Hematologic changes associated with the stress response may persist for several days after the stressor is removed [39,40]. Juvenile teleosts have notably higher lymphocyte and total leukocyte counts compared with adults [15,22].

Noninfectious diseases also can manifest in the blood of fishes; these often are associated with husbandry practices and environment. Among husbandry-related diseases, a microcytic normochromic anemia can result from environmental stressors, such as increases in population density [41,42]. Higher lymphocyte and total leukocyte counts are found in fish from production systems with high densities, marginal water quality, and often elevated bacterial load [17]. Nitrite poisoning, also known as brown blood

Table 1
Some anemias and their etiologies in teleost fishes

Etiology	Presentation	Citation
Hemorrhagic		
Bacterial		
Aeromonas sp	External/internal lesions, septicemia	Campbell and Ellis [5]
Pseudomonas sp	External/internal lesions, septicemia	Campbell and Ellis [5]
Yersinia sp	Reticulocytosis, septicemia	Tobback et al [52]
Ammonia toxicity	Microcytic normo or hypochromic	Groff and Zinkl [18]
Nutritional deficiency		
Vitamin K	Hypocoagulation, hypochromic	Groff and Zinkl [18]
Vitamin B	Hypocoagulation, hypochromic	Groff and Zinkl [18]
Inositol	Hypocoagulation, hypochromic	Groff and Zinkl [18]
Choline	Hypocoagulation, hypochromic	Groff and Zinkl [18]
Parasites		
Leech, lamprey, isopod	External lesions, pallor, macrocytic	Sinderman [66], Nair and Nair [28]
Iron deficiency	Macrocytic normo or hypochromic	Groff and Zinkl [18]
Viral (see Table 2)		
Hemolytic		
Bacterial		
Flavobacterium columnare	Fragmentation, macrocytic hypochromic	Rehulka and Minarik [54]
Aeromonas sp	Macrocytic, ± bacteremia, septicemia	Roberts and Ellis [49]
Pseudomonas sp	Macrocytic, ± bacteremia, septicemia	Roberts and Ellis [49]
Vibrio sp	Macrocytic, ± bacteremia, septicemia	Roberts and Ellis [49]
Toxins		
Nitrite	Methemoglobinemia, hypochromic	Avilez et al [29]
Mercury contamination	Macrocytic normo or hypochromic	Elahee and Bhagwant [31]
Chlorine	Heinz bodies, methemoglobinemia	Buckley [30]
Nutritional		
Folate deficiency	Pyknotic nuclei, erythroplastids, fragmentation	Plumb et al [34], Ferguson [33]
Vitamin E deficiency	Pyknotic nuclei, erythroplastids, fragmentation	Hibiya [45], Eiras [44]
Yeast excess	Poikilocytosis, microcytic hypochromic	Sanchez-Muiz et al [46]
Hemoparasites		
Trypanoplasma	Microcytic hypochromic (cryptobiosis, sleeping sickness)	Woo [37], Rowley [48]
Trypanosoma	Microcytic hypochromic	Woo [36]
Piroplasmids	Intracytoplasmic	Campbell and Ellis [5]
Hypoxia	Macrocytic normo or hypochromic	Elahee and Bhagwant [31]
Viral (see Table 2)		
Hypoplastic		
Yersiniosis (chronic)	Septicemia, kidney/splenic necrosis	Tobback et al [52]
Toxins		
Ammonia	Cell fragility, impaired erythropoiesis	Groff and Zinkl [18]
Heavy metals	Impaired erythropoiesis, low hemoglobin	Groff and Zinkl [18], Noga [3]

Table 1 (*continued*)

Etiology	Presentation	Citation
Nutritional		
Starvation	Microcytic hypochromic, abnormal nuclei	Rios et al [47]
Vitamin B12 deficiency	Normocytic hypo or normochromic	Ferguson [33]
Parasites		
Trypanoplasma	Microcytic hypochromic, impaired production (Cryptobiosis, sleeping sickness)	Woo [37], Rowley [48]
Trypanosoma	Microcytic hypochromic, impaired production	Woo [36]
Myxozoans	Normocytic hypochromic, poikilocytosis	Hoffmann and Lommel [73]
Kidney or splenic disease	Erythropoietic tissue destruction/ displacement	Campbell and Ellis [5]

disease or new tank syndrome, occurs because of incomplete nitrification of ammonium waste in closed or high-density culture situations and can result in cyanosis and hemolytic anemia [5,29]. Ammonia and heavy metal toxicoses can result in various forms of nonregenerative anemia [3,18]. Chronic exposure to cypermethrin, a synthetic pyrethroid insecticide, may cause enlargement of erythrocytes and abnormal erythrocyte morphology yielding a macrocytic anemia [43].

Nutritional disorders, such as folic acid and vitamin E deficiency or toxicosis from rancid oils and environmental pollutants, may contribute to formation of abnormal erythrocyte nuclei and erythroplastids [44,45]. Deficiencies in dietary vitamin K and B vitamins, inositol, and choline, may cause coagulation disorders resulting in hemorrhagic anemia [18]. Folate deficiency in channel catfish (*Ictalurus punctatus*) results in chronic hemolytic anemia [34,35]. Vitamin C, iron, or copper deficiency can cause

Table 2
Hematologic features of some viral diseases of teleost fishes

Disease	Host	Presentation	Citation
IHNV	Salmonids	Hemorrhagic, hypochromic, nonregenerative anemia; loss of acid-base equilibrium	Amend and Smith [58,59]
VHSV	Many species	Severe hemorrhagic and hemolytic anemia, relative monocytosis, lymphopenia, acute mortality	Egusa [62]
SVC	Cyprinids	Hemorrhagic hypochromic anemia, neutrophilia, monocytosis.	Egusa [62]
VEN	Marine species	Hemolytic anemia with prominent intraerythrocytic inclusions, typically a chronic progression	Hershberger et al [32]

microcytic hypochromic anemia [18]. Rainbow trout fed diets containing certain peroxide-producing yeasts may develop microcytic hypochromic anemia with marked poikilocytosis [46]. Vitamin C and pyridoxine deficiencies may cause leukopenia, and biotin deficiency in cyprinids may result in leukocytosis [18]. Studies of a neotropical species, *Hoplias malabaricus*, revealed that food deprivation for extended periods may result in reversible leukopenia and thrombocytopenia [47].

Inflammatory processes

Granulocytosis often is associated with inflammation in teleost and cartilaginous fishes. Monocytes occur in low numbers in a differential white blood cell count but are actively phagocytic cells in piscine fishes [48]. A monocytosis is suggestive of an inflammatory response in teleost fishes. Neutrophilia often is associated with inflammatory processes, but neutrophils are not always phagocytic. An acute neutropenia may reflect extravasion of neutrophils at a focal site of significant insult. Some reports indicate that fish eosinophils are involved in inflammatory responses but have limited phagocytic capability [48,49].

Cell-mediated abnormalities

Lymphocytosis may indicate a leukemic condition and typically are accompanied by cellular signs of degeneration, immaturity, or malignancy. Lymphocytes play an important role in humoral and cell-mediated immunity in fish [50]. Lymphocytosis may be suggestive of immunogenic stimulation, whereas lymphopenia may be suggestive of immunosuppressive conditions.

Infection-induced abnormalities

Bacterial disease

Gram-negative bacteria, such as *Aeromonas* spp and *Pseudomonas* spp, are common causes of septicemia and hemorrhagic anemia in freshwater fish [18]. *Aeromonas* spp, *Pseudomonas* ssp, and *Vibrio anguillarum* produce hemolysins and are the most common causes of hemolytic anemia in fish [18,49]. Yersiniosis of marine fish causes hemorrhagic septicemia characterized by anemia, leukocytosis, and reticulocytosis [51,52]. A severe hemorrhagic anemia caused by cold-water vibriosis (Hitra disease) was documented in juvenile Atlantic salmon (*Salmo salar*) [53]. Brook trout (*Salvelinus fontinalis*) affected by columnaris disease (*Flavobacterium columnare*) developed macrocytic hypochromic anemia with evidence of fragmented erythrocytes noted on blood smears [54]. Fig. 3 shows a gram-positive septicemia caused by *Streptococcus iniae* in a yellow tang (*Zebrasoma flavescens*). In sharks, increases in granulocytes and decreases in lymphocytes can be associated with bacterial septicemia. Leukopenia with lymphopenia or a relative neutrophilia is

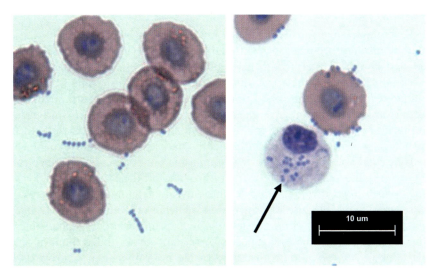

Fig. 3. Bacterial disease in a blood smear: gram-positive septicemia caused by *Streptococcus iniae*, in a yellow tang (*Zebrasoma flavescens*). Cocci are present free in the plasma and intracellularly within a neutrophil (*arrow*).

indicative of a stress response or sepsis [4,5]. Proliferative kidney disease (PKD)-affected fish are believed particularly sensitive to bacterial challenge because of the depression of granulocyte activity [55].

Viral disease

Of the myriad viral infections known from fishes, several are expressed prominently in blood, most often through the presence of intraerythrocytic inclusions or profound hemorrhagic or hemolytic anemia. Erythrocytic necrosis virus (VEN) causes hemolytic anemia and is associated with intracytoplasmic inclusions and nuclear changes in the erythrocyte of marine fish [32,56]. Erythrocytic inclusion body syndrome virus also results in intracytoplasmic inclusions but is distinct from VEN. It is associated with transient anemia in freshwater Pacific salmon in the United States but has had no adverse effects on other infected species [57]. Infectious hematopoietic necrosis virus (IHNV) infects a range of salmonid and other fish species, wherein it obliterates the lymphoid tissues of the spleen and head kidney [58,59]. Viral hemorrhagic septicemia (VHSV) has become a prominent emerging disease in the North American fisheries scene since an apparent epizootic started in the Great Lakes region in 2005 [60,61]. Spring viremia of carp (SVC) is a disease restricted to freshwater cyprinid fishes and like VHSV, it causes hemorrhagic anemia [62]. Channel catfish virus (*Herpesvirus ictaluri*) causes acute hemorrhage at the bases of the fins and in liver, kidney, and the gastrointestinal system [63,64]. Table 2 provides an overview of the clinical presentations associated with the viral diseases discussed.

Parasitic disease

Several parasites, mostly protistan, manifest in the blood of teleosts; these may be intraerythrocytic or occur in the plasma. *Trypanosoma* probably is the best-known extraerythrocytic protist in fish (Fig. 4). Fish trypanosomes essentially have the same appearance as those that cause sleeping sickness in humans (*T brucei*) and trypanosomiasis in domestic animals, although they usually are larger (example, *T mukasai* large form > 80 μm) [65] and occur at much heavier intensities than do mammalian kinetoplastids. Despite their higher parasitemia, they are infrequently pathogenic but are capable of causing fatal anemias [36]. Fish trypanoplasms are very similar in morphology to trypanosomes and are extraerythrocytic protists. *Cryptobia* (*Trypanoplasma*) *salmositica* [37] causes cryptobiosis in salmonids and may result in severe anemia because of destruction of hematopoietic tissue. *Trypanoplasma borreli* causes sleeping sickness in cyprinids with systemic illness and progressive anemia [48]. Species of trypanosomes and trypanoplasms with known life cycles are transmitted by leeches rather than arthropods.

The intraerythrocytic hemogregarines probably are the most common hemoparasites of teleosts [66,67]. Among elasmobranchs, they have been found in spiny dogfish *Squalus acanthias* [68], epaulette sharks (*Hemiscyllium ocellatum*) [69], and cat sharks (Fig. 5). Possible vectors are leeches and isopods. These usually occur as small to larger cellular inclusions in the cytoplasm of erythrocytes (see Diniz and colleagues for example [70]),

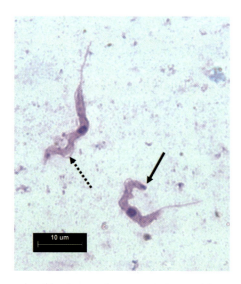

Fig. 4. Protistan disease in a blood smear: trypanosmiasis caused by an undescribed *Trypanosoma* species, in straight-backed freshwater catfish, *Neosilurus hyrtilii* from Australia. These are typical trypanosomes in possessing a recurrent flagellum that originates from a darkly staining kinetoplastid organelle (*solid arrow*) and attached to the cell by an undulating membrane (*dashed arrow*).

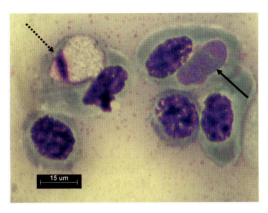

Fig. 5. Protistan disease in a blood smear: two hemogregarine morphotypes in the blood of the catshark, *Holohalaelurus punctatus.* One type (*solid arrow*) shows a fairly typical hemogregarine presentation, displacing the nucleus and with a distinct nucleus, whereas the other (*dashed arrow*) shows an unusual frothy appearance with the nucleus displaced to one pole. (*Courtesy of* Dr. Nico Smit, Department of Zoology, University of Johannesburg, South Africa.)

with or without a parasitophorous vacuole (a membrane-bound space surrounding an intracytoplasmic parasite and preventing direct contact with the cytoplasm) and with a distinct basophilic nucleus. They may appear similar to the large hemogregarines of birds and reptiles, such as *Haemoproteus*, occupying more than half of the cytoplasmic space and curving around the erythrocyte nucleus, or they may resemble the smaller, more basophilic piroplasms of mammals, such as *Babesia* spp, occurring singly or as pairs or tetrads, depending on the particular genus of parasites (see van der Straaten and colleagues for example [67]). Intraerythrocytic protist parasites of fishes (and amphibians) have been comprehensively reviewed by Davies and Johnston [71].

Many metazoan parasites cause hematologic changes, most commonly anemia, due to the consumption of host blood as part of the normal feeding biology of the parasite. They also may cause anemia by disruption of hematopoeisis. Elevated eosinophil counts are suggestive of an inflammatory response associated with antigenic stimulation or parasitic infections, such as metazoans. Leeches and lampreys are blood-sucking parasites that are large compared with most parasites and, therefore, can cause profound hemorrhagic anemia in fish. A study with captive blackeye thicklip (Labridae) showed that parasitic isopods (*Gnathia* sp) can significantly reduce hematocrit [72] as a result of the "tick-like" biology of female gnathiids, wherein they take periodic large blood meals before leaving the host to mate and molt in the substrate. Rainbow trout (*Salmo gairdneri*) affected by PKD, caused by the myxozoan parasite *Tetracapsuloides bryosalmonae*, develop a chronic normocytic hypochromic anemia with distinct poikilocytosis [73].

Thrombocytes and hemostasis

Thrombocytes play a large role in mediating the clotting response. They typically are small cells, ovoid, oblong, or spindle shaped (often all three in any given smear), with clear cytoplasm and a condensed basophilic nucleus. Some elasmobranch species have a second population of thrombocytes; in addition to the cell identical to that described for teleosts, there are thrombocytes with abundant FEGs in the cytoplasm. The clinical significance of these cells is not yet understood. Fish seem to rely primarily on extrinsic pathways of coagulation. Clot formation usually occurs within 5 minutes in teleosts whereas it may take greater than 20 minutes for some elasmobranchs to clot. Thrombocytopenia could have devastating affects on fish as not only are these cells responsible for blood clotting but also they are responsible for controlling fluid loss from surface wounds in fish. High levels of glucocorticoids decrease the number of thrombocytes and increase clotting times. Prolonged clotting times also is attributed to vitamin K deficiency [5].

Summary

Hematology of fishes lags behind that of other classes of vertebrates, but analysis of blood still can be informative about disease processes in teleosts and elasmobranchs. Although robust interpretation of fish hemograms often is hampered by a lack of reference values, this knowledge deficit represents an opportunity for expansion of clinical pathology studies among fishes. This article offers a summary of some of the more common hematologic abnormalities documented in fish and insight to some of the more obscure causes of hematologic variations and abnormalities that warrant further investigation and documentation. Practitioners are encouraged to obtain samples whenever possible as they can benefit individual animals and contribute to establishment of reference data.

References

[1] Bolasina SN. Cortisol and hematological response in Brazilian codling, *Urophycis brasilieni-sis* (Pisces, Phycidae) subjected to anesthetic treatment. Aquac Int 2006;14:569–75.

[2] Campbell TW. Tropical fish medicine. Fish cytology and hematology. Vet Clin North Am Small Anim Pract 1988;18:347–64.

[3] Noga EJ. Fish disease: diagnosis and treatment. Ames (IA): Iowa State Press; 2000.

[4] Campbell TW. Hematology of fish. In: Troy DB, editor. Veterinary hematology and clinical chemistry. Baltimore: Lippincott Williams & Wilkins; 2004. p. 277–89.

[5] Campbell T, Ellis C. Avian and exotic animal hematology and cytology. New York: Wiley-Blackwell; 2007.

[6] Fange R. Fish blood cells. In: Hoar WS, Randall DJ, Farrell AP, editors. Fish physiology, vol. 12B. San Diego (CA): Academic Press Inc; 1992. p. 1–54.

[7] Glomski CA, Tamburlin J, Chainani M. They phylogenetic odyssey of the erythrocyte. III. Fish, the lower vertebrate experience. Histol Histopathol 1992;7:501–28.

[8] Walsh CJ, Luer CA. Elasmobranch hematology: identification of cell types and practical applications. In: Smith M, Warmolts D, Thoney D, et al, editors. The elasmobranch husbandry manaual: captive care of sharks, rays and their relatives. Columbus (OH): Ohio Biological Survey, Inc; 2004. p. 307–23.

[9] Arnold JE. Hematology of the sandbar shark, *Carcharhinus plumbeus*: standardization of complete blood count techniques for elasmobranchs. Vet Clin Pathol 2005;34(2): 115–23.

[10] Lane HC. Progressive changes in hematology and tissue water of sexually mature trout, *Salmo gairdneri* Richardson during the autumn and winter. J Fish Biol 1979;34(15):425–36.

[11] Hille SA. A literature review of the blood chemistry of rainbow trout, *Salmo gairdneri* Richardson. J Fish Biol 1982;20:535–69.

[12] Ram-Bhaskar B, Srinivasa-Rao K. Influence of environmental variables on hematology, and compendium of normal hematological ranges of milkfish, *Chanos chanos* (Forskal) in brackish culture. Aquaculture 1989;83:123–36.

[13] Hrubec TC, Robertson JL, Smith SA. Effects of temperature on hematological and serum biochemical profiles of hybrid striped bass (Morone chrysops x Morone saxatilis). Am J Vet Res 1997;58(2):126–30.

[14] Hrubec TC, Robertson JL, Smith SA. Effects of ammonia and nitrate concentration on hematologic and serum biochemical profiles of hybrid striped bass (Morone chrysops × Morone saxatilis). Am J Vet Res 1997;58:131–5.

[15] Hrubec TC, Smith SA, Robertson JL. Age-related changes in hematology and plasma chemistry values of hybrid striped bass (Morone chrysops × Morone saxatilis). Vet Clin Pathol 2001;30:8–15.

[16] Valenzuela AE, Silva VM, Klempau AE. Some changes in the hematological parameters of rainbow trout *(Oncorhynchus mykiss)* exposed to three artificial photoperiod regimes. Fish Physiol Biochem 2007;33:35–48.

[17] Hrubec TC, Smith SA. Hematology of fish. In: Feldman BF, Zinkl JG, Jain NC, editors. Schalm's veterinary hematology. 5th edition. Philadelphia: Lippincott Williams & Wilkins; 2000. p. 1120–5.

[18] Groff JM, Zinkl JG. Hematology and clinical chemistry of cyprinid fish. Vet Clin North Am Exot Anim Pract 1999;2(3):741–76.

[19] Zinkle JG, Cox WT, Kono CS. Morphology and cytochemistry in leucocytes and thrombocytes of six species of fish. Comparative Hematology International 1991;1:187–95.

[20] Hine PM, Wain JM. Composition and ultrastructure of elasmobranch granulocytes. II. Rays (Rajiformes). J Fish Biol 1987;30:557–65.

[21] Hine PM, Wain JM. Composition and ultrastructure of elasmobranch granulocytes. III. Sharks (Lamniformes). J Fish Biol 1987;30:567–76.

[22] Blaxhall PC. The hematological assessment of the health of freshwater fish: a review of selected literature. J Fish Biol 1972;4:593–604.

[23] McDonald DG, Milligan CL. Chemical properties of the blood. In: Hoar WS, Randall DJ, Farrell AP, editors. Fish physiology, vol. 12B. San Diego (CA): Academic Press Inc; 1992. p. 55–133.

[24] Mylniczenko ND, Curtis EW, Wilborn RE, et al. Differences in hematocrit of blood samples obtained from two venipuncture sites in sharks. Am J Vet Res 2006;67(11):1861–4.

[25] Houston AH, Murad A. Hematological characterization of goldfish (*Carassius auratus* L) by image analysis. Effects of thermal acclimation and heat shock. Can J Zool 1991;69: 2041–7.

[26] Houston AH, Murad A. Erythrodynamics in goldfish (*Carassius auratus* L). Temperature effects. Physiol Zool 1992;65:55–76.

[27] Houston AH, Schrapp MP. Thermoacclimatory hematological response: have we been using appropriate conditions and assessment methods? Can J Zool 1994;72:1238–42.

[28] Nair GA, Nair NB. Effect of infestation with the isopod, *Alitropus typus* M. Edwards (Crustacea: Flabellifera: Aegidae) on the haematological parameters of the host fish, *Channa striatus* (Bloch). Aquaculture 1983;30:11–9.

[29] Avilez IM, Altran AE, Aguiar LH, et al. Hematological responses of the Neotropical teleost matrinxã (*Brycon cephalus*) to environmental nitrite. Comp Biochem Physiol C Toxicol Pharmacol 2004;139:135–9.

[30] Buckley JA. Heinz body hemolytic anemia in coho salmon, *Oncorhynchus kisutch*, exposed to chlorinated waste water. J Fish Res Bd Canada 1976;34:215–24.

[31] Elahee KB, Bhagwant S. Hematological and gill histopathological parameters of three tropical fish species from a polluted lagoon on the west coast of Mauritius. Ecotoxicol Environ Saf 2007;68(3):361–71.

[32] Hershberger P, Hart A, Gregg J, et al. Dynamics of viral hemorrhagic septicaemia, viral erythrocytic necrosis and ichthyophoniasis in confined juvenile Pacific herring *Clupea pallasii*. Dis Aquat Org 2006;70:201–8.

[33] Ferguson HW. Spleen, blood, lymph, thymus and reticuloendothelial system. In: Ferguson HW, editor. Systemic pathology of fish. Ames (IA): Iowa State University Press; 1989. p. 90–103.

[34] Plumb JA, Liu PR, Butterworth CE. Folate-degrading bacteria in channel catfish feeds. J Appl Aquacult 1991;1:33–43.

[35] Duncan PL, Lovell RL, Butterworth CE, et al. Dietary folate requirement determined for channel catfish, Ictalurus punctatus. J Nutr 1993;123:1888–97.

[36] Woo PTK. *Cryptobia* and cryptobiosis in fishes. Adv Parasitol 1987;26:199–237.

[37] Woo PTK. Review: *Cryptobia (Trypanoplasma) salmositica* and salmonid cryptobiosis. J Fish Dis 2003;26(11–12):627–46.

[38] Ellis AE. Bizarre forms of erythrocytes in a specimen of plaice, Pleuronectes platessa L. J Fish Dis 1984;7:411–4.

[39] Houston AH. Blood and circulation. In: Schreck C, Moyle B, editors. Methods in fish biology. Bethesda (MD): American Fisheries Society; 1990. p. 273–334.

[40] Wedemeyer GA, Barton BA, McLeay DJ. Stress and acclimation. In: Schreck C, Moyle P, editors. Methods in fish biology. Bethesda (MD): American Fisheries Society; 1990. p. 451–89.

[41] Burton CB, Murray SA. Effects of density on goldfish blood. 1. Hematology Comp Biochem Physiol A 1979;62:555–8.

[42] Murray SA, Burton CB. Effects of density on goldfish blood. 2. Cell morphology. Comp Biochem Physiol A 1979;62:559–62.

[43] Saxena KK, Seth N. Toxic effects of cypermethrin on certain hematological aspects of fresh water fish *Channa punctatus*. Bull Environ Contam Toxicol 2002;69:364–9.

[44] Eiras JC. Erythrocyte degeneration in the European eel, Anguilla anguilla. Bull Eur Assoc Fish Pathol 1985;3:8–10.

[45] Hibiya T, editor. An atlas of fish histology: normal and pathological features. Tokyo: Kodansha; 1995. p. 72–87.

[46] Sanchez-Muiz FJ, de la Higuera M, Varela G. Alterations of erythrocytes of the rainbow trout *Salmo gairdneri* by the use of *Hansenula anomola* yeast as sole protein source. Comp Biochem Physiol A 1982;72:693–6.

[47] Rios FS, Oba ET, Fernandes MN, et al. Erythrocyte senescence and hematological changes induced by startvation in the neotropical fish traíra, *Hoplias malabaricus* (Characiformes, Erythrinidae). Comp Biochem Physiol A 2005;140(3):281–7.

[48] Rowley AF. Fish. In: Rowley AF, Ratcliffe N, editors. Vertebrate blood cells. Cambridge: Cambridge University; 1988. p. 19–127.

[49] Roberts RJ, Ellis AE. The anatomy and physiology of teleosts. In: Roberts R, editor. Fish pathology. Philadelphia: WB Saunders; 2001. p. 12–54.

[50] Evans DL, Jaso-Friedmann L. Nonspecific cyto-toxic cells as effectors of immunity in fish. Annu Rev Fish Dis 1992;2:109–21.

[51] Stokes EE, Firkin BG. Studies of the peripheral blood of the Port Jackson shark (*Heterodontus portusjacksoni*) with particular reference to the thrombocyte. Br J Hematol 1971;20: 427–35.

[52] Tobback E, Decostere A, Hermans K, et al. Review: Yersinia ruckeri infections in salmonid fish. J Fish Dis 2007;30:257–68.

[53] Waagbo R, Sandness K, Espelid S, et al. Hematological and biochemical analyses of Atlantic salmon *Salmo salar* L., suffering from coldwater vibriosis ('Hitra disease'). J Fish Dis 1988; 11:417–23.

[54] Rehulka J, Minarik B. Blood parameters in brook trout *Salvelinus fontinalis* (Mitchill, 1815), affected by columnaris disease. Aquac Res 2007;38(11):1182–97.

[55] Chilmonczyk S, Monge D, deKinkelin P. Proliferative kidney disease: cellular aspects of the rainbow trout, *Oncorhynchus mykiss* (Walbaum), response to parasitic infection. J Fish Dis 2002;25(4):217–26.

[56] Wolf K. Viral erythrocytic necrosis. In: Wolf K, editor. Fish viruses and fish viral diseases. Ithica, NY: Cornell University Press; 1988. p. 389–98.

[57] Rodger HD. Erythrocytic inclusion body syndrome virus in wild Atlantic salmon, *Salmo salar* L. J Fish Dis 2007;30:411–8.

[58] Amend DF, Smith L. Pathophysiology of infectious hematopoeitic necrosis virus disease in rainbow trout (*Salmo gairdneri*): early changes in blood and aspects of immune response after injection with IHN virus. Journal of the Fisheries Research Board of Canada 1974; 31:1371–8.

[59] Amend DF, Smith L. Pathophysiology of infectious hematopoeitic necrosis virus disease in rainbow trout (*Salmo gairdneri*): hematological and blood chemical changes in moribund fish. Infect Immunity 1975;11:171–9.

[60] Řehulka J. Hematological analyses in rainbow trout *Oncorhynchus mykiss* affected by viral hemorrhagic septicaemia (VHS). Dis Aquat Org 2003;56:185–93.

[61] Lumsden JS, Morrison B, Yason C, et al. Mortality event in freshwater drum *Aplodinotus grunniens* from Lake Ontario, Canada, associated with viral hemorrhagic septicemia virus, Type IV. Dis Aquat Org 2007;76:99–111.

[62] Egusa S. Infectious diseases of fish. Tokyo: Koseisha Koseikaku Publishing; 1992.

[63] Gray WL, Williams RJ, Grin BR. Detection of channel catfish virus DNA in acutely infected channel catfish, *Ictalurus punctatus* using the polymerase chain reaction. J Fish Dis 1999;22: 111–6.

[64] Gray WL, Williams RJ, Jordan RL, et al. Detection of channel catfish virus DNA in latently infected catfish. J Gen Virol 1999;80:1817–22.

[65] Smit NJ, Van As JG, Davies AJ. Fish trypanosomes from the Okavango Delta, Botswana. Folia Parasitol 2004;51:299–303.

[66] Sindermann CJ. Principal diseases of marine fish and shellfish. San Diego (CA): Academic Press; 1990.

[67] van der Straaten N, Jacobson A, Halos D, et al. Prevalence and spatial distribution of intra-erythrocytic parasite(s) in Puget Sound rockfish (Sebastes emphaeus) from the San Juan Archipelago, Washington (USA). J Parasitol 2005;91:980–2.

[68] Clewley A, Kocan RM, Kocan AA. An intraerythrocytic parasite from the spiny dogfish, *Squalus acanthias* L., from the Pacific Northwest. J Fish Dis 2002;25(11):693–6.

[69] McKiernan JP, Grutter AS, Davies AJ. Reproductive and feeding ecology of parasitic gnathiid isopods of epaulette sharks (*Hemiscyllium ocellatum*) with consideration of their role in the transmission of a hemogregarine. International Journal for Parasitology 2005; 35:19–27.

[70] Diniz JA, Silva EO, deSouza W, et al. Some observations on the fine structure of trophozoites of the hemogregarines *Cyrilia lignieresi* (Adelina: Hemogregarinidae) in erythrocytes of the fish *Synbranchus marmoratus* (Synbranchidae). Parasitol Res 2002; 88:593–7.

[71] Davies AJ, Johnston MRL. The biology of some intraerythrocytic parasites of fishes amphibia and reptiles. Adv Parasitol 2000;45:2–109.

[72] Jones CM, Grutter AS. Parasitic isopods (*Gnathia* sp) reduce hematocrit in captive blackeye thicklip (Labridae) on the Great Barrier Reef. J Fish Biol 2005; 66:860–4.

[73] Hoffmann R, Lommel R. Hematological studies in proliferative kidney disease of rainbow trout (*Salmo gairdneri* Richardson). J Fish Dis 1984;7:323–6.

ELSEVIER
SAUNDERS

VETERINARY
CLINICS
Exotic Animal Practice

Vet Clin Exot Anim 11 (2008) 463–480

Amphibian Hematology

Matthew C. Allender, DVM, MS[a],*,
Michael M. Fry, DVM, MS,
DACVP–Clinical Pathology[b]

[a]*Department of Small Animal Clinical Sciences, College of Veterinary Medicine,
University of Tennessee, 2407 River Drive, Knoxville, TN 37996, USA*
[b]*Department of Pathobiology, College of Veterinary Medicine, University of Tennessee,
2407 River Drive, Knoxville, TN 37996, USA*

The diversity of extant amphibians comprises more than 4600 known species in three suborders of salamanders, frogs and toads, and caecilians [1]. Adult amphibians inhabit aquatic, terrestrial, and fossorial environments and have highly diverse anatomic and physiologic characteristics. Even within a given species, many intrinsic and extrinsic factors influence hematologic parameters. Hematologic reference values are rarely reported in most species, however [2]. Hematologic evaluation is nevertheless of great potential clinical value in amphibians [3,4], and many of the basic hematologic principles that apply to other vertebrates are also relevant to amphibians.

Amphibian blood is similar in many respects to reptilian and avian blood. Like reptiles and birds and unlike mammals, amphibians have nucleated erythrocytes (red blood cells [RBCs]) and thrombocytes (the word used to describe the nonmammalian equivalent of platelets). The normal color of amphibian plasma depends on the species, and it may vary from light yellow to light blue, green, or orange [5]. The similarities in blood from amphibians, reptiles, and birds may be useful to the veterinarian from a comparative standpoint so as to help understand patterns in health and disease, but major differences between mammals and nonmammalian species also pose diagnostic challenges, as discussed in more detail in this review.

Because of the wide species variability and infrequent presentation of amphibians to veterinarians, there is a paucity of information on which to base interpretation of hematology results. The authors' intent in this article is to summarize the current understanding of clinical hematology in

* Corresponding author.
E-mail address: mattallender@utk.edu (M.C. Allender).

1094-9194/08/$ - see front matter © 2008 Elsevier Inc. All rights reserved.
doi:10.1016/j.cvex.2008.03.006   *vetexotic.theclinics.com*

amphibians, emphasizing those points that are of greatest interest to veterinarians in general practice. Readers who would like a more comprehensive overview of amphibian hematology should consult other recent sources [4,5].

Natural history and environmental factors

The unique life cycle of amphibians requires an aquatic stage that involves a metamorphosis into an adult form. Some species naturally retain larval characteristics, termed *neoteny*, such as the presence of gills, which may have an impact on various hematologic values. Numerous studies have evaluated the effect of metamorphosis on hematologic values [6,7]. Controlled studies in metamorphosing individuals found a decrease in leukocyte populations, indicating susceptibility to infections [6,7]. Specifically, lymphocytes and neutrophils were demonstrated to decrease midclimax of metamorphosis [7].

Anatomic differences, such as body mass in larval salamanders, were positively correlated with some RBC indices and with blood oxygen capacity [8], providing evidence for allometric scaling.

In amphibians, temperature plays a key role in immune function. A study evaluating the effect of cold temperatures determined that long-term suboptimal temperature exposure resulted in decreases in T-lymphocyte proliferation, eosinophil numbers, and serum complement activity and an increase in neutrophils [9]. Furthermore, recent work demonstrated that temperature alterations leave individuals susceptible to infections because of the negative effects on the immune system [10]. Additionally, it has been demonstrated that elevations in altitude cause hemoconcentration and decreases in RBC volume [11].

These examples serve as a reminder that inherent individual and environmental factors other than disease processes can affect hematologic test results and should be considered when interpreting a hemogram.

Blood collection

Blood volume

Numerous factors influence the circulating blood volume in an amphibian patient, including species, season, and health status [4]. There are reports of blood volumes ranging up to 25% of body weight in caecilians, whereas several other species have reported blood volumes near 10% of body weight [4]. It is generally accepted that 10% of the blood volume can safely be removed from healthy animals without adverse effects [4]; therefore, 1% of body weight in most species (eg, 1 mL of blood from a 100-g animal) seems to be safe. Blood volume from sick or injured animals should take into account the specific disease process affecting the animal.

Animal restraint

Blood can be collected from amphibians using physical or chemical restraint. Physical restraint (Figs. 1 and 2) is preferred in most patients, especially in patients in which illness would preclude anesthesia. Amphibian integument is important to numerous body functions, including protection and respiration, and is sensitive to damage, and it is suggested to wear gloves to minimize damage. It is recommended that nonlatex gloves be used when handling amphibians because latex gloves have been proved to be lethal to larval amphibians [12]. Until further studies indicate the safety of latex gloves in adult amphibians, they should be avoided.

It is recommended to anesthetize patients when acquiring a sample by means of cardiocentesis, because small movements may damage the cardiac muscles or internal structures. General anesthesia can be accomplished using tricaine methane sulfate (most commonly) or isoflurane [13,14]. Published protocols are discussed elsewhere [4,13].

Venipuncture sites

Blood can safely be removed from several sites in an amphibian patient. In most species of frogs, venous access is gained through the ventral abdominal vein, lingual plexus, femoral vein, and heart. In addition to these sites, blood can be collected from the ventral tail vein in salamanders. Amphibians have an extensive set of lymph vessels that usually accompany blood vessels. Contamination of blood samples with lymph may lead to false

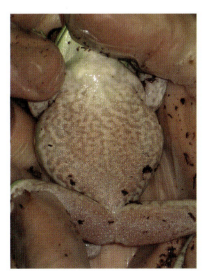

Fig. 1. Proper restraint of a White's tree frog (*Pelodryas caerulea*) for access to the ventral abdominal and femoral veins.

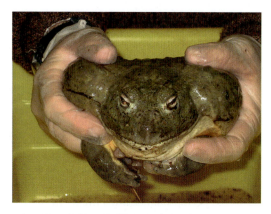

Fig. 2. Proper restraint of an African bullfrog (*Pyxiecephalus adspersus*) in preparation for venipuncture of the lingual plexus.

interpretation of anemia, or lymphocytosis. Care must be taken to avoid these lymph vessels, but clinical judgment should be used when interpreting results when lymph contamination is suspected. Some researchers recommend keeping heparinized microhematocrit tubes readily available when attempting blood collection; thus, even a small drop of blood forming on the surface of the integument can be collected by means of capillary action for analysis [4].

Venipuncture attempts at the lingual plexus can be safely used in frogs as small as 25 g [4]. Care must be taken in opening the mouth, and it is often advantageous to have an assistant hold the mouth open while venipuncture is attempted. Once the mouth is opened, the tongue is depressed to expose the buccal surface of the oral cavity. The lingual plexus is then readily visible (Fig. 3). The sample collection is collected in a 1-mL syringe with a 25-gauge

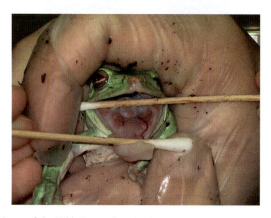

Fig. 3. Lingual plexus of the White's tree frog (*Pelodryas caerulea*), which is a common site for venipuncture in frogs and toads.

needle. Saliva may contaminate a sample taken from this plexus but may be minimized by cleaning the site with a cotton-tipped applicator before collection.

The ventral abdominal vein can be accessed between the sternum and pelvis (Fig. 4) [4]. The vein lies subcutaneously along the midline. A 25-gauge needle can be used for this site. Care must be taken not to direct dorsally into the coelom, wherein vital organs may be damaged. The femoral vein is accessed subcutaneously on the medial aspect of the hind leg. A 25-gauge needle attached to a 1-mL syringe is recommended for most amphibian patients.

In salamanders, the ventral tail vein may be used for sample collection. The vein lies ventral to the vertebrae along the midline. A 23- to 25-gauge needle attached to a 1- or 3-mL syringe is directed perpendicular to the spine.

Cardiocentesis may be performed in animals in which blood cannot be collected from other sites. It is recommended to anesthetize these patients to avoid untoward effects of collection. The heart lies near the pectoral girdle in most species but may vary with species. A 25-gauge needle is directed into the ventricle of the heart. Negative pressure in the syringe may collapse the heart; therefore, the syringe should be allowed to fill with each heart beat. It is advantageous to heparinize the syringe to avoid clotting during filling.

Sampling handling and blood smear preparation

Blood samples should be placed into anticoagulant tubes immediately after collection; ideally, a blood smear should be made before doing so. Samples that are not to be analyzed immediately should be refrigerated. Slides and blood tubes should be labeled with the animal identification and date, and relevant conditions (eg, ambient temperature, anesthesia)

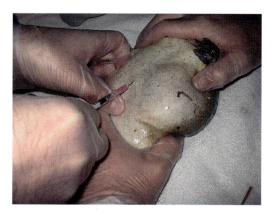

Fig. 4. Demonstration of venipuncture from the ventral abdominal vein in an African bullfrog (*Pyxiecephalus adspersus*).

should be noted in the record. Lithium heparin is the preferred anticoagulant because it seems to have minimal effect on plasma electrolyte levels and does not cause hemolysis [4,5]. A technique is described of adding sterile water to a lithium heparin tube and pretreating the syringe with that liquid before collection [4]. Alternatively, a nonheparinized syringe may be used, with blood immediately placed into the anticoagulant tube. Calcium ethylenediaminetetraacetic acid (EDTA) is not recommended because of numerous reports on the lysis of blood cells [4,15]. EDTA (dipotassium and calcium) has been avoided for reptiles for the same reason, however, and recent studies in certain reptilian species have demonstrated that EDTA may be superior for hematologic analysis [16,17].

A well-made blood smear is a key component of a complete hematologic evaluation, and a poorly made smear may severely limit the diagnostic value of a blood sample (eg, a poorly made smear may make it impossible to perform a good white blood cell [WBC] differential count). This limitation is true of samples from any species but especially so in the case of nonmammalian species in which routine automated tests are not valid. A good blood smear should not extend to the edges of the slide and should have a feathered edge. Detailed instructions for making a blood smear are available [18].

Blood smears may be made from anticoagulated blood or, preferably, from a drop of non-anticoagulated blood placed on a slide immediately after collection. Once the smear is made, it should be dried immediately. In most settings, this is easily accomplished by waving the slide in the air, but in some high-humidity settings, it may help to hold the slide in front of a hair dryer set on low (warm rather than hot). All slides should be labeled with the animal identification information and the date. In practice, blood smears are typically stained with rapid Wright type stains, such as the Camco Stain Pak (Cambridge Diagnostic Products, Ft. Lauderdale, Florida). Heparin may impart a different staining quality to some blood cells. This usually does not impede interpretation, but making a smear from a drop of fresh non-anticoagulated blood avoids the problem altogether. In general, it is advisable to use consistent laboratory methods to minimize introduced variation among samples.

Hematologic tests

The complete blood cell count (CBC), a diagnostic cornerstone in virtually every sick patient in domesticated mammals, provides basic information about the concentration and characteristics of blood cells, the plasma protein concentration, and the presence of infectious organisms in the blood. Many of the routine automated components of the CBC cannot be performed accurately on samples from nonmammalian species, however, because of problems caused by nucleated RBCs and thrombocytes. Examples of tests that are not valid in amphibians using conventional automated methods include cell counts, hemoglobin concentration, mean cell volume

(MCV), mean cell hemoglobin (MCH), and mean cell hemoglobin concentration (MCHC).

As discussed previously, other factors that may further complicate hematologic evaluation of amphibians include sample volume restrictions, contamination of blood with lymph, and poor understanding of what is normal in a given species. Despite these limitations, good hematologic data may be obtained from a small volume of amphibian blood using simple laboratory methods, which is information that may be useful in assessing an animal's current health, progression of disease, or response to therapy. An algorithm for analyzing small volumes of blood has been proposed [4]. In the authors' opinion, if only a single drop of blood is available, a blood smear would be most beneficial.

Hematologic tests that may be performed on amphibian blood with basic equipment available in most veterinary practices include the following.

Packed cell volume

This basic test is a reliable means of assessing RBC mass in amphibians provided that it is done properly and there is no significant lysis (in vitro or in vivo) of RBCs or contamination of the blood with lymph.

Blood smear examination

Preparation and staining of blood smears have been discussed previously. Microscopic examination of a stained smear is a standard means of assessing cell morphology, WBC differential counts, and presence of infectious organisms and is a subjective means of assessing cell concentrations (approximately normal, decreased, or increased).

Various formulas for estimating the concentrations of WBCs and thrombocytes from a blood smear have been proposed, none of which are extremely accurate or precise. The concentration of WBCs is commonly determined with a hemacytometer. The concentration of thrombocytes is typically assessed subjectively, and any thrombocyte clumping is noted. It has been suggested that appreciable clumping of thrombocytes indicates there is likely a sufficient concentration of them to support normal hemostasis, but it is unclear whether this rule of thumb is reliable.

Hemacytometer cell counts

The most accurate way to measure the concentration of blood cells in amphibian blood is to count the cells in a hemacytometer chamber. In principle, any cell type may be counted with a hemacytometer, and detailed techniques are described in the literature [5], but this method is used most commonly to determine the concentration of WBCs. One problem that may be encountered when examining amphibian blood is that small lymphocytes may be confused with thrombocytes. Amphibian thrombocytes often have an elongated oval to fusiform shape and have fairly abundant and almost colorless cytoplasm, whereas lymphocytes are usually round and have less abundant and more basophilic cytoplasm. Even in amphibians, however, it is easier to distinguish these two cell types on a stained blood smear than on a hemacytometer preparation.

The authors' preferred way to count nonmammalian WBCs with a hemacytometer is to use the Avian Leukopet (Vetlab Supply, Palmetto Bay, Florida) or a similar (eg, Eosinophil Unopette, Utech Products, Inc., Schenectady, New York) method, which uses a diluent that preferentially stains heterophils and eosinophils, and then to back-calculate the total WBC count based on the manual differential WBC count from the blood smear. For example, if the combined concentration of heterophils and eosinophils based on the hematocytometer count is 6500 cells/μL, and the proportions of heterophils and eosinophils based on the blood smear are 70% and 10%, respectively, the total WBC count would be calculated as follows:

$$\text{WBCs}(\#/\mu\text{L}) = \frac{\#\ \text{heterophils + eosinophils per } \mu\text{L}}{\%\ \text{of heterophils + eosinophils}}$$

$$\text{WBCs}(\#/\mu\text{L}) = (6500/0.80)$$

$$\text{WBCs}(\#/\mu\text{L}) = 8125$$

It has been suggested that this method may not work in all amphibian species and that it should be evaluated by comparing results with those obtained using Natt-Herrick's solution, which stains all cells [4].

White blood cell differential

A minimum of 100 cells are counted on a stained blood smear, and the percentages of each WBC type are then multiplied by the total WBC count (#/μL) to determine the concentrations (#/μL) of each WBC type.

Other hematologic tests that may be performed on amphibian blood using different methods than those routinely used for mammalian samples include the following.

Hemoglobin concentration

Automated hematology analyzers designed for mammalian samples provide accurate results for amphibian samples only if the RBCs are fully lysed, the sample is centrifuged, and the hemoglobin measurement is performed on the supernatant. The authors are not sure whether normal color variation of some amphibian plasma interferes with spectrophotometric measurement of hemoglobin.

Calculated mean cell volume, mean cell hemoglobin, and mean cell hemoglobin concentration values

These values require accurate values for RBC concentration and hemoglobin concentration.

Plasma protein concentration

The conventional mammalian CBC also includes a refractometer plasma protein measurement. Refractometers are calibrated based on the normal relation between refractive index and plasma protein in mammals; thus, this method may not be reliable in amphibians. Nevertheless, the test may be of some clinical value, especially to compare results of sick and healthy animals of the same species or to monitor trends in a patient over time. If an accurate plasma protein measurement is needed, the spectrophotometric (biuret) method routinely used by reference laboratories is a better choice.

Normal cell morphology and function

Red blood cells

Amphibian RBCs and thrombocytes are nucleated. The primary function of RBCs in amphibians, as in other vertebrates, is to transport oxygen by means of hemoglobin. Amphibian RBCs are oval in shape, are larger than mammalian RBCs, and have oblong nuclei with condensed chromatin and irregular margins (Fig. 5). Mean erythrocyte dimensions reported in one species of frog are 20.7 × 13.4 μm [19], mean dimensions reported in other species of frog are similar [19], and there are reports of some erythrocytes measuring up to 70 μm in diameter [5,20]. Small, round to irregular, basophilic cytoplasmic inclusions, similar to those often found incidentally in reptiles, are often found within the cytoplasm of amphibian RBCs and are considered within normal limits. Some salamanders and newts have been reported to have anucleated RBCs, including a genus of lungless salamanders in which more than 90% of RBCs lack nuclei [21], and RBCs of variable morphology have been described in some caecilians [4].

Reticulocytes (immature RBCs) may be seen occasionally as a normal finding in amphibians; the proportion of immature cells in circulation depends on the species [5]. Reticulocytes have a characteristic bluish cytoplasmic color (polychromasia) and also typically have chromatin that is less highly condensed than that of mature RBCs (see Fig. 5A). Reticulocytes in amphibians are also rounder (less ellipsoid) and smaller than mature RBCs.

White blood cells

Lymphocyte morphology in amphibians is similar to that in other species (see Fig. 5B). Lymphocytes are the predominant type of WBC in some

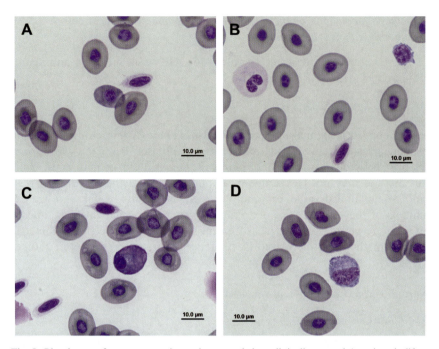

Fig. 5. Blood smear from a non-anticoagulant sample in a clinically normal American bullfrog (*Rana catesbiana*); Camco stain. (*A*) Several mature RBCs, a polychromatophilic RBC (overlapping a mature RBC in the center of the field), and a thrombocyte are noted. (*B*) Several RBCs and, clockwise from the left, a hyposegmented neutrophil, a lymphocyte, and a thrombocyte are noted. All the neutrophils in this animal were of similar hyposegmented morphology. (*C*) Several RBCs and a plasma cell are noted. (*D*) Several RBCs and a monocyte are noted.

amphibians [22,23]. As mentioned previously, small lymphocytes may be confused with thrombocytes. Furthermore, contamination of the blood sample with lymph may lead to an inaccurate interpretation of lymphocytosis. Presumably in healthy animals, most lymphocytes are small lymphocytes, and "reactive" lymphocytes responding to antigenic stimulation have more abundant cytoplasm and less condensed chromatin. It may be difficult to distinguish between large lymphocytes and monocytes [22,23]. Rare plasma cells may be noted in circulation in clinically normal animals, even in absence of lymph contamination (M.M. Fry, personal observation, 2008) (see Fig. 5C).

Granulocytes

Granulocytes in amphibians are identified based on morphologic similarities to granulocytes in other species. It is generally presumed that the function of amphibian granulocytes is similar to that of cells of similar morphology in other species; however, as has been pointed out, that may not be the case [4].

Neutrophils (heterophils)

The morphology of these cells is variable. In some species, they lack discernible cytoplasmic granules, whereas in other species, they have prominent eosinophilic granules. Those with discernible granules are often referred to as heterophils [15]. Heterophil granules are typically smaller and more elongate than those of eosinophils and may be irregularly shaped [4]. The type of stain used may also influence granulocyte morphology; at least one researcher has noted that Wright-Giemsa stain results in increased staining of basophilic granules [4]. Most amphibian neutrophils probably have lobulated nuclei, but some clinically normal amphibians may have hyposegmented neutrophils (see Fig. 5B).

Eosinophils

Amphibian eosinophils have nuclei that are usually less lobulated than those of neutrophils and intensely staining eosinophilic granules that are usually round.

Basophils

Amphibian basophils typically have intensely staining basophilic cytoplasmic granules and nuclei that are not lobulated. Degranulated basophils may also be seen in circulation, however [4]. The size of basophils relative to the size of other granulocytes varies among species [4]. Basophils are the predominant type of WBC in some amphibians [15]. Amphibian mast cells have also been described, but it not clear whether they are an entirely different lineage than basophils or a different developmental stage [4]; the clinical significance of these cells is not clear to us.

Monocytes

The morphology of monocytes in amphibians is similar to that in other species (see Fig. 5D). Some researchers have described amphibians as having azurophils in addition to, or instead of, monocytes, a distinction that, according to some, is of little clinical benefit [5]. As mentioned previously, monocytes may be confused with large lymphocytes.

Thrombocytes

These cells are considered the functional equivalent of mammalian platelets but are larger, nucleated, and usually ellipsoid (often quite elongated) to fusiform in shape (see Fig. 5A–C); some researchers state that thrombocytes become spindle shaped when activated [5]. Immature thrombocytes are round cells with round nuclei and more basophilic cytoplasm. They are rarely noted in healthy animals but are more likely than mature thrombocytes to be confused with lymphocytes.

Hematopoiesis

Erythropoiesis

There are major differences in erythropoiesis between juvenile and adult amphibians. The primary site of erythropoiesis in juvenile amphibians occurs in the liver and kidney [24–26], whereas in adults, erythropoiesis occurs in the spleen and liver in addition to the bone marrow in frogs and toads [24,25]. Thyroxine treatment influences erythropoiesis development into adult sites [25]. Erythrocytes may show differences depending on the site of production [5]. Furthermore, the hemoglobin molecule present in juveniles is distinct from hemoglobin produced in adults [27]. Therefore, changes in health status causing endocrine disruption, unnaturally delaying metamorphosis, may demonstrate an increased concentration of juvenile hemoglobin compared with adult hemoglobin. Anemia may be further differentiated based on the site of erythropoiesis. The development of an erythrocyte in *Xenopus* is reported to have the following stages: proerythroblast, erythroblast I, erythroblast II, young erythrocyte I, young erythrocyte II, and mature erythrocyte [26]. A genetic study on erythropoietin (EpoR) in *Xenopus* demonstrated genetic similarity of mammalian EpoR, and the spleen, liver, kidney, and peripheral blood were identified as sites of EpoR expression [28].

Granulopoiesis

The kidney, liver, spleen, and bone marrow are sites of granulopoiesis in most amphibians [5,26]. Aquatic species lack bone marrow. The thymus is the site of T-cell differentiation [26]. The main sites of granulopoiesis of neutrophils (bone marrow), basophils (spleen), eosinophils, and monocytes (liver) in adult *Xenopus* have been reported [26]. The development of granulocytes in *Xenopus* is reported to have the following stages: myeloblast, promyelocyte, myelocyte, metamyelocyte, band, and segment [26].

Interpretation of results

Accurately interpreting laboratory data in any species requires understanding what is normal, patterns of abnormalities in different physiologic or pathologic states, and effects of various interference on results. In amphibians, the first of these requirements often poses the greatest difficulty. Laboratory reference values should be species specific and method specific and should be based on samples acquired from high numbers of healthy individuals representing the population of interest, ideally from at least 60 clinically normal individuals [29]. Normal values not only vary among species but may be influenced by many other factors, including stage of development (larval versus adult) age, gender, reproductive status, and environmental variables (eg, wild versus captive, food and water availability, temperature, photoperiod, altitude). Understandably, hematologic reference values for amphibians are scarce and of uneven quality and are lacking altogether in most species.

In the clinical setting when reference values are available, it is helpful to know the details of the reference animal population and laboratory methods used. For cases in which reference values are unavailable or their validity is questionable, it is recommended that one or more samples from clinically normal individuals be collected as a basis for comparison. In any case, veterinarians working with amphibians must often draw on their under-standing of hematology in other animal classes. In general, conditions with abnormal blood cell concentrations or morphology are presumed to be similar in amphibians to those in other vertebrates, however, some reports have correctly pointed out that this may not necessarily be the case [4]. Some amphibians may have hematologic responses similar to those in fish, and others may have responses more similar to those in reptiles [5]. As with any species, sequential data from a given patient are likely to be helpful with monitoring progression of disease or response to therapy, and the veterinarian should integrate hematologic findings together with patient history, signs, and any other available clinical information.

Red blood cell abnormalities

An increased concentration of immature RBCs (polychromatophilic RBCs, or reticulocytes) indicates increased erythropoiesis. In anemic animals, this increase indicates a compensatory regenerative response. It is presumed that in amphibians, as in mammals, regenerative anemia usually occurs in cases of hemorrhage or hemolysis. Differential diagnoses for nonregenerative anemia in amphibians are presumed to include underlying inflammatory disease, decreased hormonal stimulation, malnutrition, neo-plasia, and bone marrow toxicity. How rapidly anemia develops in cases of decreased erythropoiesis depends on RBC life span. In some amphibians, RBC life span is greater than 100 days (as cited in an article by Wright [4]). In addition to polychromasia, morphologic features of RBCs, such as anisocytosis, hypochromasia, and poikilocytosis (RBC shape abnormali-ties), may be noted. RBC parasites are discussed in the section on disorders and diseases.

White blood cell abnormalities

The understanding of amphibian WBC responses to disease is limited. In general, however, neutrophilia (or heterophilia) and monocytosis are con-sidered consistent with inflammation; eosinophilia is considered consistent with parasitism; and lymphocytosis is considered consistent with excitement, immunologic stimulation, or lymphoid neoplasia [5]. Monocytes containing phagocytosed bacteria or other material have been described [4]. The degree to which other leukogram abnormalities recognized in other vertebrates (eg, "left shift," toxic change, stress leukogram) also occur in amphibians is not well documented. As mentioned previously, some clinically normal amphibians may have neutrophils that are not segmented (Fig. 5B). Toxic granulation of granulocytes has been recognized [4], but its clinical significance is not well characterized.

Thrombocyte abnormalities

Conditions associated with abnormal thrombocyte concentrations or morphology are presumed to be similar in amphibians and other vertebrates. An increased concentration of immature thrombocytes may suggest increased thrombopoiesis [5].

Disorders and diseases

Bacterial, fungal, and viral infections

Bacterial infections are common in captive amphibians and can be anticipated to lead to an increase in heterophils [4] and monocytes in chronic infections. Studies in *Xenopus* have elucidated the role of B lymphocytes in bacterial infections, however, and it is reported that they have phagocytic capabilities in response to these infections [30]. Phagocytic cells released from the dorsal lymph sac resulted in clearance of a *Staphylococcus* infection mediated through a peripheral increase in macrophages, a process that does not depend on temperature [6]. Treatment of infections is based on diagnosis of the pathogen with cytology and culture and sensitivity, leading to proper antimicrobial therapy, which has been discussed in other texts [4].

Hematologic responses to viral infections have rarely been documented in amphibians. One viral pathogen *Ranavirus*, caused by a member of the Iridoviridae family of viruses, has led to numerous mortality events in wild populations of frogs and salamanders [31–33]. Animals usually die before hematologic abnormalities are detected, but intracytoplasmic or intranuclear inclusions within erythrocytes may be seen [5,34]. Proliferation of T cells, specifically CD8 cells, has been indicated as a protective mechanism against Ranavirus infections [35]; therefore, lymphocytosis may be seen on a CBC.

Hematologic changes attributable to fungal infections depend on the degree and site of infection. *Saprolegnia* infections are common and presumably may lead to increases in monocytes. Infection from the well-reported chytrid fungus is restricted to the dermis and rarely cause changes in a CBC [36].

Parasitic infestations

Systemic parasite infestations uncommonly cause disease in free-ranging amphibians. In captivity, these infestations usually induce a more severe disease, often inducing eosinophilia. Furthermore, parasites may directly infest the vascular system. Nematodes of the order Filaroidea may be found in blood and lymphatic system [37]. Microfilariae infestation of these parasites causes lethargy, but severe infestation is usually required before systemic signs are seen. Treatment of these microfilariae requires removal of the intermediate host (usually insect), and treatment with fenbendazole and other anthelmintics has been suggested [38]. Erythrocytic protozoa have been reported in amphibians with a wide distribution [37]. Parasites reported in amphibians include *Haemogregarina*, *Plasmodium*, *Aegyptianella*, *Haemoproteus*, and *Lankesterella* [5,37]. Hemogregarines and *Aegyptianella* spp are common intraerythrocytic organisms considered to be of low pathogenicity; however, they have been associated with anemia in some animals, and the proportion of affected RBCs may affect prognosis [4,5]. *Bartonella ranarum* has been reported in a frog, leading to death within 6 months [37]. Extracellular hematoparasites that may be found in amphibians include trypanosomes and microfilaria, but their clinical significance is unknown [5]. Treatment of intraerythrocytic parasites is rarely necessary because their clinical significance is unknown, but parasite-specific medication may be used on a case-by-case basis [38].

Neoplasia

Hematopoietic or lymphoid neoplasia in the amphibian has been rarely reported [39]. Lymphosarcoma has been reported in the literature, but retrospective analysis of the published reports question whether these cases represent lymphosarcoma or infectious granulomas [39]. One case in the Registry of Tumors in Lower Animals demonstrates a confirmed lymphosarcoma with leukemia, but no antemortem signs were available [39]. Because of this confusion, little information is available as to the origin, clinical signs, diagnosis, and treatment of this disorder in amphibians. An extensive review of the histopathologic descriptions of hematopoietic and lymphoid neoplasia is discussed elsewhere [39].

Toxicants

Environmental toxins have been demonstrated to have a negative impact on the function of the immune system and to decrease lymphocyte counts [40]. A study evaluating the effects of toxins on circulating blood counts indicated significant differences in polluted environments, with erythrocyte fractions being most severely affected [41]. Increased mitotic erythrocytes were hypothesized because of changes in oxygen or carbon dioxide tension in polluted water [41]. Reductions in immune function facilitate opportunistic infections, with subsequent clinical signs of the pathogen isolated as discussed previously. Patients that have chronic or recurring disease may have been exposed to some of these toxins if contaminated ground water is used. Furthermore, environmental toxicants may alter circulating levels of glucocorticoids. A report showed that the presence of chemical contaminants, including exogenous glucorticoid treatment, resulted in lower eosinophil counts and increased susceptibility to parasite-induced limb deformities [42,43]. Diagnosis requires water and environmental sampling and investigation for secondary infections. Treatment of toxin exposure should follow guidelines for the specific agent identified. Noninfectious causes, such as these toxicoses, should be considered, in addition to infectious disease processes, when interpreting an abnormal amphibian hemogram.

Acknowledgments

The authors thank the keepers at the Knoxville Zoological Gardens for their assistance in restraint for blood collection.

References

[1] Pough FH. Classification and diversity of extant amphibians. In: Herpetology. New Jersey (NJ): Prentice-Hall; 1998. p. 37–74.

[2] Coppo JA, Mussart NB, Fioranelli SR. Blood and urine physiological values in farm-cultured *Rana catesbiena* in Argentina. Rev Biol Trop 2005;53:545–59.

[3] Gentz EJ. Use of amphibians in the research, laboratory, or classroom setting: medicine and surgery of amphibians. Institute for Laboratory Animal Research Journal 2007;48:255–9.

[4] Wright K. Amphibian hematology. In: Wright K, Whitaker B, editors. Amphibian medicine and captive husbandry. Malabar (FL): Krieger Publishing; 2001. p. 129–46.

[5] Campbell TW, Ellis CK. Hematology of amphibians. In: Avian and exotic animal hematology and cytology. Ames (IA): Blackwell Publishing; 2007. p. 83–91.

[6] Kolias GV. Immunologic aspects of infectious diseases. In: Hoff G, Frye F, Jaconson E, editors. Diseases of amphibians and reptiles. New York: Plenum Press; 1984. p. 661–91.

[7] Ussing AP, Rosenkilde P. Effect of induced metamorphosis on the immune system of the Axotyl, *Ambyostoma mexicanum*. Gen Comp Endocrinol 1995;97:308–19.

[8] Burggren WW, Dupre RK, Wood SC. Allometry of red cell oxygen binding and hematology in larvae of the salamander, *Ambystoma tigrinum*. Respir Physiol 1987;70:73–84.

[9] Maniero GD, Carey C. Changes in selected aspects of immune function in the leopard frog, *Rana pipiens*, associated with exposure to cold. J Comp Physiol [B] 1997;167: 256–63.

[10] Raffel TR, Rohr JR, Kiesecker JM, et al. Negative effects of changing temperature on amphibian immunity under field conditions. Functional Ecology 2006;20:819–28.

[11] Biswas HM, Boral MC. Changes of body fluid and hematology in toad and their rehabilitation following intermittent exposure to simulated high altitude. Int J Biometeorol 1986;30: 189–97.

[12] Sobotka JM, Rahwan RG. Lethal effect of latex gloves on *Xenopus laevis* tadpoles. J Pharmacol Toxciol Methods 1994;32:59.

[13] Stetter M. Amphibians. In: West G, Heard D, Caulkett N, editors. Zoo animal and wildlife immobilization and anesthesia. Ames (IA): Blackwell Publishing; 2007. p. 205–9.

[14] Wright K. Restraint techniques and euthanasia. In: Wright K, Whitaker B, editors. Amphibian medicine and captive husbandry. Malabar (FL): Krieger Publishing; 2001. p. 111–22.

[15] Campbell TW. Hematology of amphibians. In: Thrall MA, editor. Veterinary hematology and clinical chemistry. Philadelphia: Lippincott, Williams & Wilkins; 2004. p. 291–7.

[16] Hanley CS, Hernandez-Divers SJ, Bush S, et al. Comparison of the effect of dipotassium ethylenediaminetetraacetic acid and lithium heparin on hematologic values in the green iguana (*Iguana iguana*). J Zoo Wildl Med 2004;35:328–32.

[17] Mayer J, Knoll J, Innis C, et al. Characterizing the hematologic and plasma chemistry profiles of captive Chinese water dragons, *Physignathus cocincinus*. Journal of Herpetological Medicine and Surgery 2005;15:45–52.

[18] Harvey JW. Atlas of veterinary hematology: blood and bone marrow of domestic animals. Philadelphia: Saunders; 2001. p. 8–9.

[19] Singh K. Hematology of the common Indian frog (*Rana tigrina*). I. Erythrocytes. Anat Anz 1977;141(3):280–4.

[20] Pessier AP. Cytologic diagnosis of disease in amphibians. Vet Clin North Am Exot Anim Pract 2007;10:187–206.

[21] Scott RB. Comparative hematology: the phylogeny of the erythrocyte. Blut 1966;12: 340–51.

[22] Cathers T, Lewbart GA, Correa M, et al. Serum chemistry and hematology values for anesthetized American bullfrogs (*Rana catesbeiana*). J Zoo Wildl Med 1997;28(2):171–4.

[23] Singh K. Hematology of the common Indian frog (*Rana tigrina*). II. Leucocytes. Anat Anz 1977;141(5):445–9.

[24] Tanaka Y. Architecture of the marrow vasculature in three amphibian species and its significance in hematopoietic development. Am J Anat 1976;145:485–98.

[25] Maniatis GM, Ingram VM. Erythropoiesis during amphibian metamorphosis: site of maturation of erythrocytes in *Rana catesbeiana*. J Cell Biol 1971;49:372–9.

[26] Hadji-Azimi I, Coosemans V, Canicatti C. Atlas of Xenopus laevis laevis hematology. Dev Comp Immunol 1987;11:807–74.

[27] Maniatis GM, Ingram VM. Erythropoiesis during amphibian metamorphosis: immunolochemical detection of tadpole and frog hemoglobins (*Rana catesbeiana*) in single erythrocytes. J Cell Biol 1971;49:380–9.

[28] Yergeau DA, Schmerer M, Kuliyev E, et al. Cloning and expression pattern of the Xenopus erythropoietin receptor. Gene Expr Patterns 2006;6:420–5.

[29] Stockham SL, Scott MA. Fundamentals of veterinary clinical pathology. Ames (IA): Iowa State Press; 2002. p. 11.

[30] Li J, Barreda DR, Zhang Y-A, et al. B lymphocytes from early vertebrates have potent phagocytic and microbicidal abilities. Nat Immunol 2006;7:1116–24.

[31] Green DE, Converse KA, Schrader AK. Epizootiology of sixty-four amphibian morbidity and mortality events in the USA, 1996–2001. Ann N Y Acad Sci 2002;969:323–39.

[32] Bollinger TK, Mao J, Schock D, et al. Pathology, isolation, characterization of a novel iridovirus from tiger salamanders in Saskatchewan. J Wildl Dis 1999;35:413–29.

[33] Jancovich JK, Mao J, Chichar G, et al. Genomic sequence of a ranavirus (family *Iridoviridae*) associated with salamander mortalities in North America. Virology 2003; 316:90–103.

[34] Speare R, Freeland WJ, Bolton SJ. A possible iridovirus in erythrocytes of *Bufo marinus* in Costa Rica. J Wildl Dis 1991;27:457–62.

[35] Morales HD, Robert J. Characterization of primary and memory CD8 T-cell responses against ranavirus (FV3) in *Xenopus laevis*. J Virol 2007;81:2240–8.

[36] Pessier AP, Nichols DK, Longcore JE, et al. Cutaneous chytridiomycosis in poison dart frogs (*Dendrobates* spp.) and White's tree frogs (*Litoria caerulea*). J Vet Diagn Invest 1999;11:194–9.

[37] Reichenbach-Klinke H, Elkan E. Infectious diseases. In: The principle diseases of lower vertebrates. New York: Academic Press; 1965. p. 220–320.

[38] Poynton SL, Whitaker BR. Protozoa and metazoan infecting amphibians. In: Wright K, Whitaker B, editors. Amphibian medicine and captive husbandry. Malabar (FL): Krieger Publishing; 2001. p. 193–221.

[39] Green DE, Harshbarger JC. Spontaneous neoplasia in amphibia. In: Wright K, Whitaker B, editors. Amphibian medicine and captive husbandry. Malabar (FL): Krieger Publishing; 2001. p. 335–400.

[40] Christin M-S, Gendron AD, Brousseau P, et al. Effects of agricultural pesticides on the immune system of *Rana pipiens* and on its resistance to parasitic infection. Environ Toxicol Chem 2003;22:1127–33.

[41] Barni S, Boncompagni E, Grosso A, et al. Evaluation of *Rana* snk *esculenta* blood cell response to chemical stressors in the environment during the larval and adult phases. Aquat Toxicol 2007;81:45–54.

[42] Belden LK, Kiesecker JM. Glucocorticosteroid hormone treatment of larval treefrogs increases infection by *Alaria* Sp. trematode cercariae. J Parasitol 2005;91:686–8.

[43] Kiesecker JM. Synergism between trematode infection and pesticide exposure: a link to amphibian limb deformities in nature? Proc Natl Acad Sci U S A 2002;99:9900–4.

ELSEVIER
SAUNDERS

VETERINARY
CLINICS
Exotic Animal Practice

Vet Clin Exot Anim 11 (2008) 481–500

Reptile Hematology

John M. Sykes IV, DVM, DACZM[a],*,
Eric Klaphake, DVM, DACZM, DABVP–Avian[b,c]

[a]*Gottlieb Animal Health and Conservation Center, Los Angeles Zoo,
5333 Zoo Drive, Los Angeles, CA 90027, USA*
[b]*ZooMontana, 2100 South Shiloh Road, Billings, MT 59106, USA*
[c]*Animal Medical Center, 216 North 8th Avenue, Bozeman, MT 59715, USA*

The basic principles of hematology used in mammalian medicine can be applied to reptiles. This article outlines techniques for sample collection, processing, and analysis that are unique to reptiles and provides a review of factors influencing interpretation of the results.

Restraint and blood collection techniques

General comments

Before collecting a blood sample, the maximum safe volume that can be collected should be determined. Reptiles have a lower total blood volume compared with a similarly sized mammal, 5% to 8% of their body weight [1,2], and 10% of this volume may be safely collected from healthy reptiles (eg, 0.5–0.8 mL in a 100-g animal). Smaller samples should be collected from compromised individuals.

Lithium heparin is generally the anticoagulant of choice in reptiles, because ethylenediaminetetraacetic acid (EDTA) has been reported to cause hemolysis, particularly in chelonians [3,4]. Other studies of multiple reptilian species suggest that EDTA produces comparable or better quality blood smears than those using heparin, however [5–8]. Hematology slides should be prepared from uncoagulated samples immediately after collection to avoid complications related to the anticoagulant. A study of slide preparation using blood obtained from green iguanas (*Iguana iguana*) [9] found that the coverslip slide method and bevel-edge slide techniques were adequate in

* Corresponding author.
E-mail address: john.sykes@lacity.org (J.M. Sykes).

producing quality smears, whereas the slide-slide method produced lower quality smears (higher numbers of ruptured cells). Slides are stained with a Romanowsky type stain for morphologic analysis (eg, Giemsa, Wright, Wright-Giemsa) [10,11]. Rapid stains, such as Diff-Quik, may result in understaining or damage to some cell types [11].

Snakes

There are two common venipuncture sites in snakes: the caudal tail vein and the heart [12,13]. For either site, proper restraint of the snake's head is critical for handler safety. The caudal tail vein is accessed by holding the snake in dorsal recumbency and stabilizing the tail caudal to the cloaca. Holding the tail ventral to the body, such as over the end of a table, aids in successful collection. The needle is inserted on the midline between one third to one half of the distance from the cloaca to the tip of the tail (usually 6–12 scutes caudal to the cloaca) at an angle of 45° directed cranially. Avoid puncture of the hemipenes and scent glands, which lie on either side of the midline. The needle is advanced with slight negative pressure. If vertebrae are encountered, the needle should be backed out and redirected. Restraint for this site is easy, but risks include lymphatic contamination, trauma, or infection to the hemipenes or scent glands, and it is difficult to collect a large volume. This site is useful for larger snakes and rattlesnakes but is often more difficult to access in some colubrids and smaller boids.

For direct cardiac puncture, the snake is restrained in dorsal recumbency. The heart is usually located one fourth to one third of the distance from the head to the tail [12,14]. It is found by visual inspection, palpation, or, occasionally, an ultrasound probe, particularly in larger snakes. Stabilize the heart with a finger cranial and the thumb caudal to the heart, taking care not to apply too much pressure, which may occlude blood flow in and out of the heart (Fig. 1). The needle is inserted at an angle of 45° into the ventricle of the heart. The syringe fills slowly with each heart beat using only minimal negative pressure. Moderate digital pressure for up to 1 minute after needle withdrawal can decrease hematoma formation [12]. This technique can be performed safely in nonsedated snakes with adequate restraint, provided that the needle is minimally moved when in the body. If redirection is required, the needle should be withdrawn to the skin, redirected, and then advanced again.

Venipuncture of the palatine vein of snakes [15] is not recommended because of difficulties in restraint, minimal blood flow, and significant hematoma formation.

Lizards

Blood collection in lizards is usually from the tail vein, with the lizard restrained in ventral or dorsal recumbency. Species that perform tail autotomy

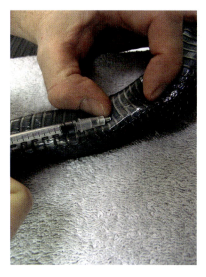

Fig. 1. Cardiac puncture for blood collection from a snake.

may need to be anesthetized (eg, with intramuscular ketamine) [16] before using this technique. One may also use the vagal technique (for calming lizards) by applying pressure over both eyes digitally or by taping cotton balls over closed eyes. The tail vein can be accessed ventrally or laterally. The ventral approach is performed as described previously for snakes. For the lateral approach, the needle is inserted at an angle of 90° to the tail, just ventral to the lateral processes of the vertebrae, and directed medially. This site is identified by the longitudinal groove in which the dorsal and ventral musculature meet, although the groove can be difficult to locate in obese individuals.

The ventral abdominal vein lies within the coelomic cavity just dorsal to the ventral midline between the umbilicus and sternum. The lizard must be well restrained or anesthetized in dorsal recumbency, and the needle should be inserted along the ventral midline at a shallow angle and directed cranially. There is a risk for lacerating the vessel without the ability to apply pressure after the procedure, and puncture of other visceral structures is possible [12,17].

Chelonians

Many venipuncture sites for chelonians have been described, including the heart; jugular, subcarapacial, femoral, brachial, and coccygeal veins; and occipital sinus [12,18,19]. The optimal site varies with the size and species, sedation level, medical condition, and experience of the phlebotomist. Samples collected from the jugular vein may be least likely to result in hemodilution, because the vein can be visualized [20]. Regardless of site, pressure should be applied after collection for hemostasis.

The subcarapacial site is useful and easy to access in many species, particularly if access to the neck or limbs is difficult [18,21]. The head and neck can be in extension or withdrawn into the shell. The needle is inserted on the midline, where the skin of the neck meets the carapace. The exact angle of the needle to the body varies with the shape of the carapace but is advanced along the ventral aspect of the carapace using mild negative pressure (Fig. 2) [21]. This site is the preferred alternative to toenail clipping for nonmedical personnel [22].

Although the jugular vein may be preferred, it is accompanied by difficult restraint. The chelonian is positioned in ventral recumbency with the head held in a slightly more "head-down" position and with pressure applied to the back legs. The head is grasped using a ventral approach to avoid the normal defensive retraction response to dorsal threats. Grasping an extended foreleg prevents hinged tortoises from "boxing up." Do not forcibly extract the head using instruments to avoid significant trauma to the beak. Once the head is restrained and extended, the vein is raised and visualized by applying pressure laterally at the thoracic inlet, digitally or using a cotton-tipped applicator in smaller individuals.

The presence and location of coccygeal veins in chelonians vary by species and may be dorsal, lateral, or ventral [12]. The dorsal vein can be accessed by flexing the tail ventrally and inserting the needle in a cranioventral direction as far cranially as possible on the dorsal midline. Lateral and ventral veins may be accessed in a similar technique to that previously described for lizards, but quantity may be limited.

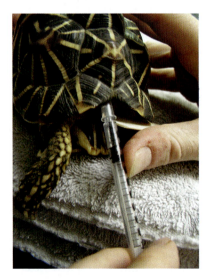

Fig. 2. Blood collection from the subcarpacial vein of a tortoise.

The brachial vein (also called brachial plexus or ulnar plexus) [18] is located near the tendon of the triceps at the radiohumeral joint (elbow) [19]. The foreleg is grasped and extended. The triceps tendon is palpated near the caudal aspect of the elbow joint, and the needle is inserted ventral to the tendon with the syringe held parallel to the forearm (Fig. 3). Aldabra tortoises (*Geochelone gigantean*) have been trained for voluntary blood collection at this site [23]. Quantity collected may be limited.

Cardiocentesis may be performed if other sites are not available but is generally reserved for administration of euthanasia solution [18,19]. A needle is placed directly through the plastron on the midline near the junction of the pectoral and abdominal scutes [12,19]. An access hole may need to be drilled through the plastron before inserting the needle, which is sealed with epoxy or dental acrylic after collection [10]. Access by means of the thoracic inlet is difficult because of the inability to stabilize the heart and the required needle length [19].

Two different approaches to the occipital sinus have been described [19,24]. In sternal recumbency, extend the head, aim the nose ventrally, and then direct the needle caudally on the dorsal midline of neck just caudal to occiput [19]. Alternatively, position the chelonian vertically, extending and then flexing head to make an angle of 90° with the shell, and cranially direct the needle into the sinus at the dorsal midline of the neck [24]. With either method, a 25- or 23-gauge needle is used and adequate manual or chemical restraint is critical.

The dorsal cervical sinuses (lateral occipital sinuses) are unique to sea turtles [18]. The turtle is restrained in sternal recumbency with the head flexed ventrally. The sinuses are dorsal and lateral to the cervical vertebrae. The needle is directed at up to an angle of 90° into the sinus. These sinuses cannot be palpated and may be fairly deep. Neck-restraining boxes or use of an ultrasound machine may help to locate the proper site in larger sea turtles (Fig. 4).

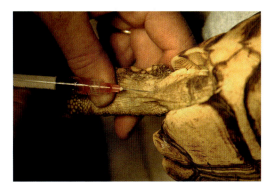

Fig. 3. Blood collection from the brachial vein of a box turtle (*Terrapene carolina carolina*).

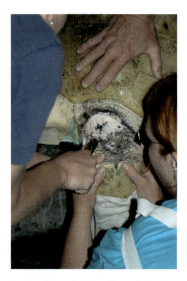

Fig. 4. Blood collection from the lateral cervical sinuses of a sea turtle.

Crocodilians

The ventral tail vein and the supravertebral sinus are the most commonly used sites in crocodilians. The ventral tail vein is accessed as in snakes. The supravertebral sinus is accessed by restraining the animal in ventral recumbency with the head controlled. The needle is placed on the ventral dorsal midline just caudal to the occiput and directed ventrally at an angle of 90° (Fig. 5). Spinal cord trauma can occur if needle is advanced too deeply [12].

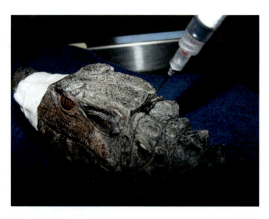

Fig. 5. Blood collection from the occipital sinus of a crocodilian.

Bone marrow collection

Marrow can be collected from the femur or tibia of most lizards, crocodilians, and chelonians as in mammals [12]. In chelonians, marrow may also be obtained from between the outer and inner layers of bony shell [10]. The outer keratin is drilled through, and marrow is then aspirated from between the layers. In snakes, a rib biopsy is the most reliable method to obtain marrow [10,12]. An entire rib is surgically removed, and marrow is then aspirated, or the rib can be submitted in formalin for histopathologic evaluation. Place an encircling ligature proximal to the transaction site to prevent bleeding of intercostal vessels.

Sample analysis

Erythrocytes

The packed cell volume (PCV), total erythrocyte count (RBC), and erythrocyte morphology should always be evaluated [11,13]. The PCV can be measured using hematocrit tubes as for mammals. The total RBC can be obtained using automated cell counters or manually [25]. Manual methods involve a hemocytometer and some type of staining or dilution system. The erythrocyte Unopette (Becton-Dickinson, Rutherford, New Jersey) is one such system; an alternative system uses Natt and Herrick's solution and a diluting pipette. Use of the Natt and Herrick solution allows determination of the RBC and total leukocyte count (WBC) using the same sample in the hemocytometer [10].

Mature reptilian erythrocytes are oval with an irregularly margined nucleus (Figs. 6–10) [10,11,26]. New erythrocytes are created from the bone marrow; extramedullary sites, such as the liver and spleen; or mature circulating cells dividing to form daughter cells [10]. Thus, mitotic figures in circulating reptile erythrocytes may be normal. Compared with mature erythrocytes, immature cells appear smaller and more round, have a basophilic cytoplasm, and have less dense chromatin in the nucleus (Fig. 11) [11]. Reticulocytes can be observed using a new methylene blue stain and are 2.5% or less of the normal total RBC [11]. Hemoglobin, mean cell volume, and mean cell hemoglobin concentration are calculated as for mammals.

Leukocytes

Complete leukocyte analysis includes a WBC, differential, and morphologic assessment [11,13]. Because of the nucleated nature of reptile erythrocytes, automated methods of obtaining a WBC and differentials are not accurate. Manual methods for obtaining a WBC include estimated counts from blood smears, the semidirect method with phloxine B solution (eg, Unopette system), and the direct method (eg, using Natt and Herrick's solution). Each method has advantages and disadvantages, and the accuracy of results depends on the cytologist's experience.

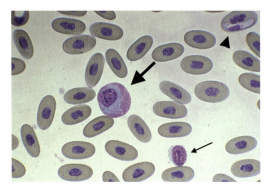

Fig. 6. Erythrocytes, azurophil (*large arrow*), and small lymphocyte (*small arrow*) of a yellow rat snake (*Elaphe obsolete quadrivittata*). One erythrocyte (*arrowhead*) has an intracellular Haemogregarina parasite (EDTA, aqueous Romanowsky's stain, original magnification ×330). (*Courtesy of* Ed Ramsay, DVM, DACZM, Knoxville, TN.)

The estimated count method is performed by counting the total number of leukocytes in at least 10 fields of a stained blood smear using the high-dry (×40 or ×45) objective. The average number of leukocytes per field is multiplied by 1500, resulting in the estimated number of leukocytes per microliter. This method is rapid and simple but is prone to error if cells are clumped or not evenly distributed on the slide [27].

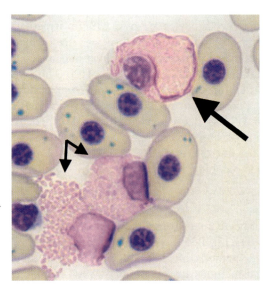

Fig. 7. Erythrocytes, heterophil (*large arrow*), and two eosinophils (*small arrows*) of a freshwater turtle (*Hieremys annandalii*). Intracytoplasmic inclusions of the erythrocytes are attributed to artifact (lithium heparin, Romanowsky's stain, original magnification ×1000). (*Courtesy of* Adrienne Adkins, DVM, Gainesville, FL.)

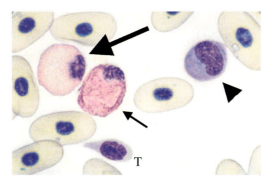

Fig. 8. Erythrocytes, heterophil (*large arrow*), eosinophil (*small arrow*), azurophilic monocyte (*arrowhead*), and thrombocyte (T) of a freshwater turtle (*Deirochelys reticularia*). Intracytoplasmic inclusions of the erythrocytes are attributed to artifact (lithium heparin, Romanowsky's stain, original magnification ×1000). (*Courtesy of* Adrienne Adkins, DVM, Gainesville, FL.)

The semidirect method is performed by staining acidophilic granulocytes with phloxine B solution. These stained granulocytes are counted in a hemocytometer, and a differential cell count is performed on a stained slide. The total WBC is then calculated using the number of heterophils and eosinophils counted in the hemocytometer and the percent of such cells on the differential: Total WBC/μL = Number of Cells Stained in Hemocytometer Chamber × 1.1 × 16 × 100/Percentage of Heterophils and Eosinophils on Differential [25,28]. This method requires an accurate differential for calculation of the WBC. If the heterophil count is low (because of true heteropenia or lysis of heterophils during creation of the blood smear), the total WBC can be artificially elevated.

The direct method is performed by staining all leukocytes with a solution, such as Natt and Herrick's; the leukocytes are counted using

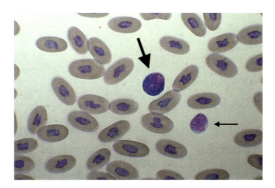

Fig. 9. Basophil (*large arrow*) and small lymphocyte (*small arrow*) of a yellow rat snake (*Elaphe obsolete quadrivittata*) (EDTA, aqueous Romanowsky's stain, original magnification ×330). (*Courtesy of* Ed Ramsay, DVM, DACZM, Knoxville, TN.)

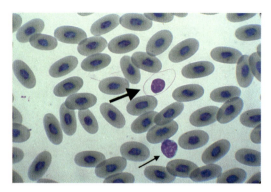

Fig. 10. Thrombocyte (*large arrow*) and lymphocyte (*small arrow*) of a yellow rat snake (*Elaphe obsolete quadrivittata*) (EDTA, aqueous Romanowsky's stain, original magnification ×330). (*Courtesy of* Ed Ramsay, DVM, DACZM, Knoxville, TN.)

a hemocytometer, and the total WBC is calculated. This method relies on distinguishing small lymphocytes from thrombocytes in the hemocytometer [11,29]. Inaccurately counting thrombocytes as lymphocytes artificially elevates the result.

Heterophils (see Figs. 7 and 8) are the most common granulocyte in reptile blood and are analogous to the neutrophil [10,13]. They are round, may have pseudopodia, and have clear cytoplasm [10,13]. The nucleus is round and eccentric and may be bilobed [13,29]. The granules are eosinophilic, elongated, or spindle shaped and may be numerous [11,29]. The morphology of heterophils may vary within an individual, particularly in the staining qualities of the granules. This variation has been hypothesized to be attributable to different stages of maturation of the heterophil, because this cell may mature while in circulation [30–32]. Toxic changes may be represented by the presence of a basophilic cytoplasm, abnormal granules, and vacuoles [29,33].

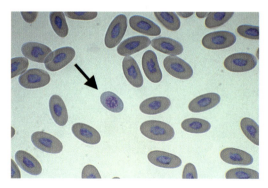

Fig. 11. Immature erythrocyte (*arrow*) of a yellow rat snake (*Elaphe obsolete quadrivittata*) (EDTA, aqueous Romanowsky's stain, original magnification ×330). (*Courtesy of* Ed Ramsay, DVM, DACZM, Knoxville, TN.)

Eosinophils (see Figs. 7 and 8) are of similar size and shape to heterophils, and an eccentric nucleus is present. The distinguishing morphologic feature is that the eosinophilic granules of eosinophils are usually spherical rather than the oval or elongated granules of heterophils [10,11,29]. Eosinophils of green iguanas (*I iguana*) are unusual because of their bluish-green spherical granules, the function of which is unknown [34]. Eosinophils are not present in all species, particularly in snakes [13]. They have been found in king cobras (*Ophiophagus Hannah*) [32] but not in diamondback rattlesnakes (*Crotalus adamanteus*) [30] or yellow rat snakes (*Elaphae obsoleta quadrivitatta*) [8]. Variation of eosinophils within individuals, as described for heterophils, has been observed in green turtles (*Chelonia mydas*) [35].

Basophils (see Fig. 9) are small granulocytes with darkly basophilic granules that obscure the centrally located nonlobed nucleus [10,11]. Care should be taken to distinguish between a normal basophil and a toxic heterophil, in which granules are basophilic and round [29].

Lymphocytes (see Figs. 6, 9, and 10) of reptiles are morphologically similar to those of mammals. They lack granules, may be small or large, have a high nucleus-to-cytoplasm ratio, and have basophilic cytoplasm [11,26]. These cells may have phagocytosed particles or erythrocytes [10,29]. They typically contour to the shape of adjacent cells [8,29].

Monocytes (see Fig. 8) are also similar to those of mammals. They are often the largest leukocyte (species dependent), with a variably shaped contour and nucleus [11,13]. Monocytes of many nonsquamate reptiles contain azurophilic granules. These cells may be reported as "azurophils" or "azurophilic monocytes" but are a variation of the normal monocyte rather than a distinct cell type [11,34]. In contrast, azurophils of snakes (see Fig. 6) are a distinct cell type whose function is similar to the neutrophil [30]. The azurophils of snakes have finer granules and round nuclei compared with the azurophilic monocytes of other reptiles, which have coarser granules and a lobulated nucleus [36].

Thrombocytes (see Figs. 8 and 10) are small oval basophilic cells with a central basophilic nucleus and pale blue or colorless cytoplasm [10,11]. It is important to distinguish between small lymphocytes and thrombocytes when performing differential counts or using the direct method of obtaining the total WBC. Small lymphocytes are more round, with darker cytoplasm and more clumped chromatin in their nuclei when compared with thrombocytes [13,29].

Factors affecting the hemogram

Demographic factors

Species, slide staining and evaluation technique, health status, nutritional status, age, reproductive status, stress levels, gender, venipuncture site, season, hibernation status, captivity status, and environmental factors can affect the values and the presentation of blood cells.

In interpreting these effects, differentiate between statistically significant variation and clinically relevant variation. Do not extrapolate demographic variations beyond species and settings described in a study. The findings of several recent studies are described here to demonstrate the complexity in evaluating reptilian hemograms when such factors are taken into consideration.

In Mediterranean pond turtles (*Mauremys leprosa*), the leukocyte differential of free-ranging animals did not follow the pattern previously described for captive *M leprosa*, in which the percentage of lymphocytes ranged between 64.9% and 57.8% in captive animals compared with 4.2% and 7.7% in free-ranging turtles. A similar leukocyte differential from another fresh water turtle (*Emys orbicularis*) sampled in the same locality suggested the influence of environmental factors in the study area as a cause of the lower lymphocyte percentages [37].

In northern red-bellied cooters (*Pseudomys rubriventris*), age and species variation were noted. Hematocrit values were lower for turtles from one of three institutions studied in which younger animals were present, consistent with findings reported in box turtles (*Terrapene carolina*). As in other species of freshwater turtles, but not other chelonians, basophils were the most predominant leukocyte in *P rubriventris* [38].

Nesting female leatherback turtles (*Dermochelys coriacea*) had lower eosinophil percentages compared with green (*C mydas*) and loggerhead turtles (*Caretta caretta*). This was attributed to lower helminth parasite loads in leatherbacks because of their diet of jellyfish. In addition, the WBC count based on the eosinophil Unopette method (2800–5900 cells/μL) compared with slide estimation (1600–4500 cells/μL) was statistically different ($P \leq .05$) in this study [39].

Although a study of viperid snakes found no differences between pre- and posthibernation values [40], seasonal differences for nonhibernating species have been noted. Twenty-five captive adult boa constrictors (*Boa constrictor amarali*) had significant differences ($P \leq .05$) in RBC, WBC, lymphocyte, thrombocyte, and monocyte counts based on season, demonstrating the importance of the period of the year in the interpretation of reference values in these animals. A significant increase in heterophil, eosinophil, basophil, and lymphocyte concentrations has been observed in other reptiles during summer, followed by a reduction in winter [41]. Whole blood collected in January and August from 18 captive radiated tortoises (*Geochelone radiata*) found RBC and PCV values significantly higher in summer versus winter and higher in male tortoises versus female tortoises. These differences were attributed to vitellogenesis in female tortoises and altered hydration status and activity in summer [42]. Environmental temperature variation, along with more age-related variation, was noted in western fence lizards (*Sceloporus occidentalis*), in which the hematocrit was higher at 15° versus 30°C and lower in hatchling lizards [43].

Another factor to consider is immobilization or restraint of the reptiles. Stress was induced in 99 captive estuarine crocodiles (*Crocodylus porosus*) by two different handling methods: manual restraint (noosing with ropes) and immobilization by electrostunning. The study found that the stress response of stunned animals, as measured by increases in PCV and hemoglobin, was significantly reduced compared with that of manually restrained crocodiles. Both groups showed a significant increase in PCV and hemoglobin concentration; however, the magnitude of change was significantly reduced and recovery was faster in stunned animals [44].

Lymphodilution

Because lymphatic vessels and sinuses usually run in tandem with veins, lymphodilution can occur with any sample. Even cardiocentesis can have contamination or dilution with pericardial fluid. Contamination is recognized by a quick filling of clear fluid into the syringe, followed by blood. Removal of some of the lymph in a particular venipuncture site before withdrawal of the needle may result in a "cleaner" sample on the next venipuncture attempt. This phenomenon may be attributable to collapse of the weak-walled lymphatic vessel (or pericardial space), allowing the needle to push through to the vein or heart, although this is purely conjecture. Grossly contaminated samples are easily recognized and should be discarded. In other situations, however, the hypothetical questions to be asked are as follows:

1. How does one know if there is lymphatic contamination in clinically insignificant amounts?
2. How much contamination is required to cause clinically relevant changes in the hemogram?

One method to address these questions is to measure the PCV of the sample immediately after collection. If less than 10%, the sample should be discarded (unless severe anemia is clinically feasible) and redrawn. In small, critical, or dangerous reptiles, this may not be an option, but the validity of the interpretation of the hemogram should be questioned (and may not be worth the client's money) if the sample is extremely diluted.

Disorders of hematology

Much of what is written regarding the interpretation of reptilian hematologic results and their causes is anecdotal and based on mammalian assumptions. Association of cause with diagnostic results and correct treatment is often lacking in the peer-reviewed literature, because many thorough cases usually include necropsy and histopathology to make for a stronger case report. What follows are personal anecdotal observations combined with reports from the literature when applicable.

Erythrocytic disorders

Anemia

The diagnosis of anemia may be artifactual, based on amount of hemodilution present, and some reptiles have normally low PCV ranges, such as 16% to 21% in ball pythons (*Python regius*) [45]. Thus, interpretation of anemia must be made carefully. True anemia is categorized as being attributable to blood loss, destruction, or decreased production. In many cases, a thorough history can suggest whether acute blood loss occurred, such as from trauma. Polychromasia and increased reticulocyte counts may be noted, depending on the time frame, but reptile RBCs are long-lived; thus, response is muted in comparison to mammals or birds. Anemia attributable to decreased production from chronic disease is the most common cause seen by the authors. Often, these reptiles are described as having been debilitated for weeks to months. Causes may include infection, chronic exposure to improper environment and diet, chronic organ failure (usually renal or hepatic), gastrointestinal disease, or neoplasia. Because reptiles rely on aerobic and anaerobic respiration and have a low metabolism normally, the clinical presentation of even severe anemia is difficult to assess. Mucous membranes of many reptiles may be pigmented, pale, or muddy, even in healthy specimens, and most sick reptiles are lethargic regardless of cause.

Polycythemia

Polycythemia has been suggested when the PCV exceeds 40% [11]. One author (EK) has had several cases of reptiles with PCVs of this level and higher, many with concurrent elevations of total proteins or solids. Tentative diagnosis of dehydration has been made in these individuals, often subclinical, but polycythemia has also been noted in healthy reproductively active female iguanas (E. Klaphake, personal observation, 2008).

Inclusions

Erythrocyte inclusion bodies may be attributable to artifact from staining (see Figs. 7 and 8), viral particles, or the presence of hemoparasites (see Fig. 6).

Iridovirus-related inclusion bodies have been observed incidentally and as causes of anemia in reptiles. In a fer-de-lance (*Bothrops moojeni*) evaluated for renal carcinoma, erythrocytes contained two types of inclusions, one viral and one crystalline, usually concomitantly. The snake was markedly anemic and exhibited a strong regenerative response. Ultrastructural analysis identified the virus to be an iridovirus consistent with snake erythrocyte virus and the crystalline structures to be of a different nature than hemoglobin [46]. Inclusions of viral particles consistent with iridovirus have also been found in the erythrocytes and erythroblasts of free-ranging northern water snakes (*Nerodia sipedon sipedon*) from Canada [47] and free-ranging flap-necked chameleons (*Chamaeleo dilepis*) from Tanzania [48].

The presence of hemoparasites has often been noted in nonclinical captive animals, leading to questions of their significance in captive reptiles [49]. Several free-ranging snakes in Florida inhabited the same environment with distinctive *Hepatozoon* species characteristic of each host species, none of which had apparent clinical signs [50]. There are, however, reports of pathologic findings attributable to hemoparasites. For example, blood cell composition (percent of immature erythrocytes) and blood hemoglobin were altered by infection with *Plasmodium* spp (severity varied depending on species of parasite) in eastern Caribbean island anoles (*Anolis sabanus*). Substantial data on two other lizard-malaria systems, *Sceloporus occidentalis* infected with *Plasmodium mexicanum* in northern California and *Agama agama* infected with *Plasmodium giganteum* and *Plasmodium agamae* in Sierra Leone, showed that malaria was virulent in those two associations as well [51]. Another report of a wild-caught adult female southern water snake suggested that the animal did not adjust well to captivity, in part attributable to a heavy burden of hemogregarines [52]. Fortunately, because many hemoparasites require an invertebrate as part of its life cycle, captive-raised reptiles, unless housed outdoors, seem to be at low risk for infection by these parasites.

Leukocytic disorders

Infection is a challenging diagnosis to make in reptiles based on a leukogram. Leukopenia, leukocytosis, and even a normal leukogram can all be present during infection. Even determining what defines those categories (ie, what absolute numbers meet the definitions for each species) can be challenging. Established normal values are often based on limited populations and rarely then take into account the aforementioned demographic factors. Looking for other signs, such as "toxic" cells or the distribution (ie, 90% heterophils) can also be debated by the best cytologists as to appropriate interpretation. In birds, one author (EK) uses plasma protein electrophoresis (EPH) in combination with the total WBC and distribution to make such distinctions, but in reptiles, EPH interpretation is still in its infancy and of truly unknown significance.

Leukocytosis

As mentioned previously, leukocytosis in reptiles is often associated anecdotally with infection. One author (EK) uses a WBC greater than 30,000 cells/μL to define leukocytosis in evaluating for possible infection and response. As with anemia, many illnesses in reptiles are attributable to chronic disease, wherein the WBC would be expected to have regressed back into a normal or leukopenic range through the weeks or months before presentation. Reptilian monocytosis often is observed in immune responses to bacterial infections and parasitic infestations that result in tissue granuloma formation [53].

Documented cases of leukocytosis have also been reported to be attributable to neoplastic leukemias. Hematopoietic malignancies are most commonly reported in lizards [54] and snakes [55], occurring sporadically in other reptiles. These neoplasias may present as multiple discrete masses, such as with lymphosarcoma, circulating neoplasms (leukemia), or a combination of both forms [53,56,57]. They typically occur as sporadic cases, but outbreaks or clusters of lymphoid neoplasms have been reported [58]. Determining the cell type of these neoplasms has been challenging, because standard mammalian cytochemical stains may or may not be informative [54,56].

Leukopenia

Leukopenia attributable to toxicosis associated with fenbendazole was noted in a 125-day study of Hermann's tortoises (*Testudo hermanni*). Serial blood samples found that although the tortoises remained healthy, an extended heteropenia occurred. The investigator suggested that the risk for mortality of an individual from nematode infection should be assessed relative to the potential for metabolic alteration and secondary septicemia after damage to hematopoietic and gastrointestinal systems by fenbendazole [59].

A treatment regimen for severe leukopenia was attempted in the case of a severely traumatized juvenile green sea turtle. The animal had an initial calculated total leukocyte count of 0 cells/μL and no mature circulating heterophils on the differential. The turtle was treated with antibiotics and recombinant human granulocyte colony-stimulating factor (hG-CSF) in an attempt to increase heterophil production and possibly activation. Three daily doses of hG-CSF at 6.7 μg/kg given subcutaneously resulted in a rapid increase in acidophilic progranulocytes, which subsequently declined over the next 3 days. A second regimen, consisting of a repeat of the first three-dose daily regimen followed by continued dosing every 48 hours for an additional 9 days, maintained a white blood cell count of 11,600 to 24,700 cells/μL. Three weeks after initiating therapy, mature heterophils began to appear in the peripheral blood and the hG-CSF was discontinued. Finally, after all other medications were discontinued, a 3-day regimen of hG-CSF at 6.7 μg/kg resulted in marked increases in total leukocytes, heterophils, lymphocytes, and monocytes [60]. This treatment option may warrant further evaluation in reptiles in the future and is of mention for being outside the circle of commonly considered modalities.

Inclusions and hemoparasites

As with erythrocytic inclusions, the differentials of artifact, virus, and hemoparasite should be considered. A free-ranging adult female eastern box turtle (*T carolina*) had intracytoplasmic inclusions consistent with iridovirus within heterophils and large mononuclear leukocytes on routine blood smear examination [61]. In a report of blood films examined from 170 specimens of 15 *Chamaeleo* spp in Tanzania, 3 *Chamaeleo dilepis* had an intracytoplasmic inclusion within monocytes. One of the lizards was maintained in captivity, and at 46 days, a second type of inclusion was occasionally seen within monocytes. Transmission electron microscopic examination of monocytes revealed the presence of a chlamydia-like organism and pox-like virus [62].

Thrombocytic disorders

No reports of thrombocytic disorders could be found in an extensive review of the literature or have been noted in either author's own personal experience.

Acknowledgments

The authors acknowledge the generous donation of multiple hematology figures by Drs. Ed Ramsay and Adrienne Adkins and several phlebotomy pictures taken by Noah Lindgren. Thanks to Tad Motoyama for assistance with figure preparation.

References

[1] Lillywhite HB, Smits AW. Lability of blood volume in snakes and its relation to activity and temperature. J Exp Biol 1984;110:267–74.

[2] Smits AW, Kozubowski MM. Partitioning of body fluids and cardiovascular responses to circulatory hypovolemia in the turtle *Pseudemys scripta elegans*. J Exp Biol 1985;116:237–50.

[3] Jacobson ER. Blood collection techniques in reptiles. In: Fowler ME, editor. Zoo and wild animal medicine, current therapy 3. Philadelphia: WB Saunders Co; 1993. p. 144–52.

[4] Muro J, Cuenca R, Pastor J, et al. Effects of lithium heparin and tripotassium EDTA on hematologic values of Hermann's tortoises (Testudo hermanni). J Zoo Wildl Med 1998;29(1):40–4.

[5] Harr KE, Raskin RE, Heard DJ. Temporal effects of 3 commonly used anticoagulants on hematologic and biochemical variables in blood samples from macaws and Burmese pythons. Vet Clin Pathol 2005;34(4):383–8.

[6] Hanley CS, Hernandez-Divers SJ, Bush S, et al. Comparison of the effect of dipotassium ethylenediaminetetraacetic acid and lithium heparin on hematologic values in the green iguana (*Iguana iguana*). J Zoo Wildl Med 2004;35(3):328–32.

[7] Martinez-Jimenez D, Hernandez-Divers SJ, Floyd TM, et al. Comparison of the effects of dipotassium ethylenediaminetetraacetic acid and lithium heparin on hematologic values in yellow-blotched map turtles, Braptemys flavimaculata. Journal of Herpetological Medicine and Surgery 2007;17(2):36–41.

[8] Dotson TK, Ramsay ER, Bounous DI. A color atlas of blood cells of the yellow rat snake. Compendium on Continuing Education for the Practicing Veterinarian 1995;17:1013–6.

[9] Perpinan D, Hernandez-Divers SM, McBride M, et al. Comparison of three different techniques to produce blood smears from green iguanas, Iguana iguana. Journal of Herpetological Medicine and Surgery 2006;16(3):99–101.

[10] Frye FL. Hematology as applies to clinical reptile medicine. In: Frye FL, editor. Biomedical and surgical aspects of captive reptile husbandry. 2nd edition. Malabar (FL): Krieger Publishing Co; 1991. p. 209–79.

[11] Campbell TW. Clinical pathology of reptiles. In: Mader DR, editor. Reptile medicine and surgery. 2nd edition. St. Louis (MO): Saunders; 2006. p. 453–70.

[12] Hernandez-Divers SJ. Diagnostic techniques. In: Mader DR, editor. Reptile medicine and surgery. 2nd edition. St. Louis (MO): Saunders; 2006. p. 490–532.

[13] Strik NI, Alleman AR, Harr KE. Circulating inflammatory cells. In: Jacobson ER, editor. Infectious diseases and pathology of reptiles color atlas and text. Boca Raton (FL): CRC Press; 2007. p. 167–218.

[14] Jacobson ER. Overview of reptile biology, anatomy, and histology. In: Jacobson ER, editor. Infectious diseases and pathology of reptiles color atlas and text. Boca Raton (FL): CRC Press; 2007. p. 1–130.

[15] Olson GA, Hessler JR, Faith RE. Techniques for blood collection and intravascular infusions of reptiles. Lab Anim Sci 1975;25:783–6.

[16] Schumacher J, Yelen T. Anesthesia and analgesia. In: Mader DR, editor. Reptile medicine and surgery. 2nd edition. St. Louis (MO): Saunders; 2006. p. 442–52.

[17] Redrobe S, MacDonald J. Sample collection and clinical pathology of reptiles. Veterinary Clin North Am Exot Anim Pract 1999;2(3):709–30.

[18] Barrows MS, McAurthur S, Wilkinson R. Diagnostics. In: McArthur S, Wilkinson R, Meyer J, editors. Medicine and surgery of tortoises and turtles. Oxford: Blackwell Publishing Ltd; 2004. p. 109–40.

[19] Lloyd M, Morris P. Chelonian venipuncture techniques. Bulletin of the Association of Reptile and Amphibian Veterinarians 1999;9(1):26–8.

[20] Gottdenker NL, Jacobson ER. Effect of venipuncture sites on hematologic and clinical biochemical values in desert tortoises (Gopherus agassizzi). Am J Vet Res 1995;56:19–21.

[21] Hernandez-Divers SM, Hernandaz-Divers SJ, Wyneken J. Angiographic, anatomic and clinical technique descriptions of a subcarapacial venipuncture site for chelonians. Journal of Herpetological Medicine and Surgery 2002;21(2):32–7.

[22] Johnson JD. Nail trimming for blood collection from desert tortoises, Gopherus agassizii: panel summary. Journal of Herpetological Medicine and Surgery 2006;16(2):61–2.

[23] Weiss W, Willson S. The use of classical and operant conditioning in training Aldabra tortoises (Geochelone gigantean) for venipuncture and other husbandry issues. J Appl Anim Welf Sci 2003;6(1):33–8.

[24] Martinez-Silvestre A, Perpinan D, Marco I, et al. Venipuncture technique of the occipital venous sinus in freshwater aquatic turtles. Journal of Herpetological Medicine and Surgery 2002;12(4):31–2.

[25] Pierson FW. Laboratory techniques for avian hematology. In: Feldman BF, Zinkl JG, Jain NC, editors. Schalm's veterinary hematology. 5th edition. Philadelphia: Lippincott Williams and Wilkins; 2000. p. 1145–7.

[26] Saint Girons MC. Morphology of the circulating blood cell. In: Gans C, Parsons TC, editors. Biology of the reptilia, vol. 3. New York: Academic Press; 1970. p. 73–91.

[27] Latimer KS, Bienzle D. Determination and interpretation of the avian leukogram. In: Feldman BF, Zinkl JG, Jain NC, editors. Schalm's veterinary hematology. 5th edition. Philadelphia: Lippincott Williams and Wilkins; 2000. p. 417–32.

[28] Campbell TW. Avian hematology. In: Avian hematology and cytology. Ames (IA): Iowa State University Press; 1988. p. 3–17.

[29] Wilkinson R. Clinical pathology. In: McArthur S, Wilkinson R, Meyer J, editors. Medicine and surgery of tortoises and turtles. Oxford: Blackwell Publishing Ltd; 2004. p. 141–86.

[30] Alleman AR, Jacobson ER, Raskin RE. Morphological, cytochemical staining, and ultrastructural characteristics of blood cells from eastern diamondback rattlesnakes (Crotalus adamaneus). Am J Vet Res 1999;60:507–14.

[31] Bounous DI, Dotson TK, Brooks RL, et al. Cytochemical staining and ultrastructural characteristics of peripheral blood leucocytes from the yellow rat snake (Elaphe obsolete quadrivitatta). Comparative Haematology International 1996;6:86–91.

[32] Salakiji C, Salakij J, Apibal S, et al. Hematology, morphology, cytochemical staining, and ultrastructural characteristics of blood cells in king cobras (Ophiophagus hannah). Vet Clin Pathol 2002;31(3):116–26.

[33] LeBlanc CJ, Heatley JJ, Mack EB. A review of the morphology of lizard leukocytes with a discussion of the clinical differentiation of bearded dragon, *Pogonavitticeps*, leukocytes. Journal of Herpetological Medicine and Surgery 2000;19(2):27–30.

[34] Harr KE, Alleman AR, Dennis PM, et al. Morphologic and cytochemical characteristics of blood cells and hematologic and plasma biochemical reference ranges in green iguanas. J Am Vet Med Assoc 2001;218(6):915–21.

[35] Work TM, Raskin RE, Balazs GH, et al. Morphological and cytochemical characteristics of blood cells from Hawaiian green turtles. Am J Vet Res 1998;59:1252–7.

[36] Alleman AR, Jacobson ER, Raskin RE. Morphologic and cytochemical characteristics of blood cells from the desert tortoise (*Gopherus agassizii*). Am J Vet Res 1992;53:1645–51.

[37] Hidalgo-Vila J, Diaz-Paniagua C, Perez-Santigosa N, et al. Hematologic and biochemical reference intervals of free-living Mediterranean pond turtles (*Mauremys leprosa*). J Wildl Dis 2007;43(4):798–801.

[38] Innis CJ, Tlusty M, Wunn D. Hematologic and plasma biochemical analysis of juvenile head-started northern red-bellied cooters (*Pseudemys rubriventris*). J Zoo Wildl Med 2007; 38(3):425–32.

[39] Deem SL, Dierenfeld ES, Sounguet GP, et al. Blood values in free-ranging nesting leather-back sea turtles (*Dermochelys coriacea*) on the coast of the Republic of Gabon. J Zoo Wildl Med 2006;37(4):464–71.

[40] Dutton CJ, Taylor PA. Comparison between pre- and posthibernation morphometry, hematology, and blood chemistry in viperid snakes. J Zoo Wildl Med 2003;34(1):53–8.

[41] Machado CC, Silva LFN, Ramos PRR, et al. Seasonal influence on hematologic values and hemoglobin electrophoresis in Brazilian *Boa constrictor amarali*. J Zoo Wildl Med 2006; 37(4):487–91.

[42] Zaias J, Norton T, Fickel A, et al. Biochemical and hematologic values for 18 clinically healthy radiated tortoises (*Geochelone radiata*) on St. Catherine's Island, Georgia. Vet Clin Pathol 2006;35(3):321–5.

[43] Dunlap KD. Ontogeny and scaling of hematocrit and blood viscosity in Western Fence Lizards, Sceloporus occidentalis. Copeia 2006;2006(3):535–8.

[44] Franklin CE, Davis BM, Peucker SK, et al. Comparison of stress induced by manual restraint and immobilisation in the estuarine crocodile, Crocodylus porosus. J Exp Zoolog A Comp Exp Biol 2003;298(2):86–92.

[45] Johnson JH, Benson PA. Laboratory reference values for a group of captive Ball Pythons (*Python regius*). Am J Vet Res 1996;57(9):1304–7.

[46] Johnsrude JD, Raskin RE, Hoge AY, et al. Intraerythrocytic inclusions associated with iridoviral infection in a fer de lance (*Bothrops moojeni*) snake. Vet Pathol 1997;34(3): 235–8.

[47] Smith TG, Desser SS, Hong H. Morphology, ultrastructure and taxonomic status of *Toddia* sp. in northern water snakes (Nerodia sipedon sipedon) from Ontario, Canada. J Wildl Dis 1994;30(2):169–75.

[48] Telford SR, Jacobson ER. Lizard erythrocytic virus in East-African chameleons. J Wildl Dis 1993;29(1):57–63.

[49] Campbell TW. Hemoparasites. In: Mader DR, editor. Reptile medicine and surgery. 2nd edition. St. Louis (MO): Elsevier; 2006. p. 801–5.

[50] Telford SR, Wozniak EJ, Butler JF. Haemogregarine specificity in two communities of Florida snakes, with descriptions of six new species of Hepatozoon (Apicomplexa: Hepato-zoidae) and a possible species of Haemogregarina (Apicomplexa: Haemogregarinidae). J Parasitol 2001;87(4):890–905.

[51] Schall JJ, Staats CM. Virulence of lizard malaria: three species of Plasmodium infecting *Anolis sabanus*, the endemic anole of Saba, Netherlands Antilles. Copeia 2002;2002(1):39–43.

[52] Wozniak EJ, Telford SR, DeNardo DF, et al. Granulomatous hepatitis associated with Hep-atozoon sp. meronts in a southern water snake (*Nerodia fasciata pictiventris*). J Zoo Wildl Med 1998;29(1):68–71.

[53] Gregory CR, Latimer KS, Fontenot DK, et al. Chronic monocytic leukemia in an Inland Bearded Dragon, Pogona vitticeps. Journal of Herpetological Medicine and Surgery 2004; 14(2):12–6.

[54] Hernandez-Divers SM, Orcutt CJ, Stahl SJ, et al. Lymphoma in lizards—three case reports. Journal of Herpetological Medicine and Surgery 2003;13(1):14–21.

[55] Garner MM, Hernandez-Divers SM, Raymond JT. Reptile neoplasia: a retrospective study of case submissions to a specialty diagnostic service. Veterinary Clin North Am Exot Anim Pract 2004;7(3):653–71.

[56] Tocidlowski ME, McNamara PL, Wojcieszyn JW. Myelogenous leukemia in a bearded dragon (Acanthodraco vitticeps). J Zoo Wildl Med 2001;32(1):90–5.

[57] Schultze AE, Mason GL, Clyde VL. Lymphosarcoma with leukemic blood profile in a Savannah monitor lizard (Varanus exanthematicus). J Zoo Wildl Med 1999;30(1):158–64.

[58] Gyimesi ZS, Garner MM, Burns RB, et al. High incidence of lymphoid neoplasia in a colony of Egyptian spiny-tailed lizards (Uromastyx aegyptius). J Zoo Wildl Med 2005;36(1):103–10.

[59] Neiffer DL, Lydick D, Burks K, et al. Hematologic and plasma biochemical changes associated with fenbendazole administration in Hermann's tortoises (Testudo hermanni). J Zoo Wildl Med 2005;36(4):661–72.

[60] Howard L, Rhinehart BA, Manire CA, et al. Use of human granulocyte colony-stimulating factor in a Green Sea Turtle, Chelonia mydas. J Herp Med Surg 2003;13(3):10–4.

[61] Allender MC, Fry MM, Irizarry AR, et al. Intracytoplasmic inclusions in circulating leukocytes from an eastern box turtle (Terrapene carolina carolina) with iridoviral infection. J Wildl Dis 2006;42(3):677–84.

[62] Jacobson ER, Telford SR. Chlamydial and poxvirus infections of circulating monocytes of a flap-necked chameleon (Chamaeleo dilepis). J Wildl Dis 1990;26:572–7.

VETERINARY
CLINICS
Exotic Animal Practice

Vet Clin Exot Anim 11 (2008) 501–522

Avian Hematology and Related Disorders

Elizabeth B. Mitchell, DVM, MA[a],*,
Jennifer Johns, DVM, DACVP–Clinical Pathology[b]

[a]*Companion Avian and Exotic Pet Medicine, Veterinary Medical Teaching Hospital,
University of California-Davis, One Shields Avenue, Davis, CA 95616, USA*
[b]*Department of Pathology, Microbiology, and Immunology, School of Veterinary Medicine,
University of California-Davis, One Shields Avenue, Davis, CA 95616, USA*

Hematology is an essential component of veterinary practice. The interpretation of avian blood cells provides many challenges. Practitioners must be able to recognize normal morphology and function of cells to interpret changes in those cells. This article describes the normal morphology of avian erythrocytes, leukocytes, and thrombocytes. Changes observed in erythrocytes and leukocytes during disease and major differential diagnoses are discussed. A brief overview of avian blood parasites is also presented.

There are important considerations in the preparation of avian blood smears. Small blood volume, the potential for hemolysis of erythrocytes in ethylenediaminetetraacetic acid (EDTA) anticoagulant in certain species of birds, variations in staining with traditional Wright's or Giemsa stains, and fragility of avian red blood cells (RBCs) in the preparation of smears all complicate determination of avian hematology parameters. Detailed discussions of collection and handling of blood samples have been published previously [1–5]. Therefore, these topics are not covered in detail in this review.

Avian erythrocytes and related disorders

Avian erythrocytes are nucleated elliptic cells with elliptic and centrally placed nuclei. The mature avian erythrocyte is larger than that of most mammals but smaller than those of reptiles and amphibians [1]. With

---

* Corresponding author. Veterinary Medical Teaching Hospital, School of Veterinary Medicine, University of California-Davis, One Shields Avenue, Davis, CA 95616.
E-mail address: emitchell@ucdavis.edu (E.B. Mitchell).

Wright's staining or other Romanowsky stains, the cytoplasm of the mature erythrocyte stains orange, whereas the nucleus stains dark purple. Nuclear chromatin becomes increasingly condensed with erythrocyte maturity. More immature avian erythrocytes are round cells with basophilic cytoplasm, round nuclei, and more open nuclear chromatin; elliptic erythrocytes develop approximately at the reticulocyte or polychromatophil stage (Fig. 1).

Total erythrocyte concentration, packed cell volume (PCV), and hemoglobin concentration may be influenced by age, gender, hormones, and other factors. PCV and total erythrocyte count tend to be higher in male birds than in female birds and also tend to increase with age [6]. The normal PCV for many bird species ranges approximately between 35% and 55% [7]. Avian erythrocytes have a shorter half-life, ranging from roughly 25 to 45 days in various species, than that of many mammals. Because erythrocyte turnover is more rapid, birds tend to have higher percentages of polychromatophils in health than mammals. Avian erythropoietin is a glycoprotein that is synthesized in the kidneys and stimulates bone marrow erythropoiesis. There is apparently no cross-reactivity between avian and mammalian erythropoietin [6].

Avian erythrocyte size has been reported to vary with species [8]. In a group of healthy adult psittacines, the range of calculated erythrocyte mean cell volumes (MCVs) was approximately 116 to 219 fL (Johns, unpublished data, 2006). Several erythrocyte parameters, including RBC count, may be measured quantitatively on impedance-based or flow cytometric hematology analyzers with appropriate adjustments for other nucleated

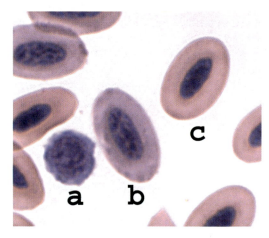

Fig. 1. Different stages of maturation of avian erythrocytes. The cell labeled ''a'' is a more immature erythrocyte. This cell is round, with a round nucleus, less densely packed nuclear chromatin, and basophilic cytoplasm. The cell labeled ''b'' is a polychromatophilic erythrocyte, as evidenced by the more basophilic cytoplasm and the elliptic shape of the cell. The cell labeled ''c'' is a normal mature avian erythrocyte, characterized by elliptic shape, purple-staining centrally located nucleus, and orange staining cytoplasm.

cells. Manual methods of counting avian erythrocytes are well described, however, and are often implemented in practice, given the paucity of automated instrumentation appropriate for use in avian hematology. The PCV can easily be obtained by means of centrifugation of a filled microhematocrit tube. Hemocytometer counting of erythrocytes can be accomplished using the Unopette (Becton-Dickinson, Rutherford, New Jersey) method or using Natt and Herrick's solution [9].

A substantial amount of information can be gained by examining a well-made blood smear. Erythrocyte morphology, including size variation (anisocytosis), shape abnormalities (poikilocytosis), and abnormalities in hemoglobinization, can be evaluated in the monolayer region of the smear. Semiquantitative estimates of polychromasia, anisocytosis, poikilocytosis, and degree of erythrocyte parasitism (if present) can be performed. A slight degree of polychromasia is common in healthy birds; one reference interval for healthy psittacines reports that polychromatophils comprised 0.41% to 6.78% of all erythrocytes [10]. Slight anisocytosis is also considered an unremarkable finding in birds [1]. Prominent anisocytosis may be seen with regenerative anemia or with dyserythropoiesis, however, and was seen in blood smears from marine birds exposed to crude oil [11].

Polychromasia (polychromatophilia) is defined as increased affinity for acidic and basic stains, and in avian erythrocytes, it is seen as increased cytoplasmic basophilia resulting in lavender- to gray-staining cytoplasm with Wright's staining. Polychromatophilic erythrocytes are often evaluated semiquantitatively in routine avian blood smears on a 1+ to 4+ scale, with 4+ polychromasia defined as greater than 30 polychromatophils per ×1000 monolayer field [7]. Polychromatophils in Wright-stained smears are considered to be roughly equivalent to reticulocytes in supravitally stained smears. Avian reticulocytes are defined by means of specific morphologic criteria, because it has been shown that a high percentage of avian erythrocytes contains basophilic granular material ("reticulum") when supravitally stained (Fig. 2) [7,12]. This granular material is present in a perinuclear ring in immature erythroid cells; as cells mature, the reticulum first disperses into scattered cytoplasmic aggregates and then diminishes and becomes punctate in appearance [13]. When avian reticulocytes (defined as having aggregates of reticulum forming a ring [contiguous or discontiguous] around at least half of the erythrocyte nucleus in total) were counted in new methylene blue–stained blood smears, the percentage of reticulocytes strongly correlated with percentage of polychromatophils in samples from a variety of avian species [10]. In the same comparison, reticulocyte percentage also proved to be a more precise value than polychromatophil percentage. Either measurement may therefore be used as an index of erythroid regenerative capacity in birds. Erythroid cells more immature than reticulocytes are round and smaller than reticulocytes or mature erythrocytes, with deeply basophilic cytoplasm. Increases in more immature erythrocytes have been seen with marked regenerative responses in birds. Lead

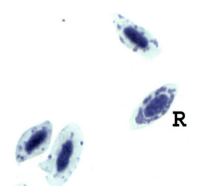

Fig. 2. Avian blood smear stained with new methylene blue stain. The cell labeled "R" is a reticulocyte, defined by the presence of an aggregate of reticulum in a ring form that surrounds at least half of the nucleus.

poisoning of birds can cause an increase in more immature erythrocytes without evidence of anemia [1].

Hypochromasia, or decreased amount of staining hemoglobin in an erythrocyte, is associated with several disease conditions in birds, including acute blood loss and inflammation [14]. Hypochromasia in mammalian erythrocytes is a finding commonly linked to iron deficiency and poorly regenerative anemia, and similar findings have been reported in birds [1]. Inflammation causes redistribution of body iron stores, reducing iron available for erythropoiesis and resulting in functional iron deficiency. Acute blood loss and nutritional iron deficiency can cause hypochromic, poorly regenerative, or nonregenerative anemia in birds because of absolute iron deficiency. Hypochromasia is also reported with lead and zinc toxicosis in birds. Experimentally induced hemolytic anemia attributable to zinc toxicosis in mallards resulted in poorly regenerative anemia with high percentages of hypochromic cells in birds that died or were euthanized as a result of severe clinical disease [14]. Poikilocytosis, particularly fusiform erythrocytes, and erythrocyte nuclear abnormalities were also prominent in this group of birds. In contrast, surviving birds had an increased percentage of polychromatophils, indicating a regenerative anemia, and significantly lower levels of poikilocytosis. The impaired regenerative response in the more severely affected birds suggests functional iron deficiency as a cause of decreased erythropoiesis and is compatible with evidence in birds and mammals that excess ingested zinc impairs iron absorption and use [15,16]. Zinc and lead toxicosis can cause regenerative hemolytic anemia, impaired heme synthesis, hypochromasia, and a shortened erythrocyte life span in birds, although one clinical report suggests that hemolysis does not occur in zinc-intoxicated birds [14,17]. In early lead toxicosis, hypochromic erythrocytes are described as having cytoplasmic ballooning, sometimes described as "D cells" when eccentric (Fig. 3) [14,18].

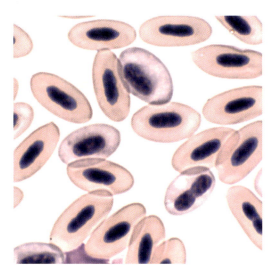

Fig. 3. Normal avian erythrocytes surround three hypochromic avian erythrocytes that are demonstrating cytoplasmic ballooning, also referred to as "D cells." The cells have decreased staining intensity, central pallor, and eccentrically placed nuclei. Cytoplasmic ballooning is commonly seen in early lead toxicosis.

Nuclear abnormalities in avian erythrocytes are usually attributable to dyserythropoiesis but occasionally occur because of markedly accelerated erythrocyte production [14]. Nuclear abnormalities can include nuclear fragmentation or pyknosis, Howell-Jolly bodies, nuclear shape changes, and binucleation. Binucleated erythrocytes are rarely reported in blood smears from normal birds, but the presence of higher numbers of binucleated cells is considered abnormal [1]. Chronic lead toxicosis can also result in nuclear abnormalities, including pyknosis within smaller senescent erythrocytes [1].

Basophilic stippling of the cytoplasm can be seen in avian erythrocytes stained with Wright's stain. As is the case with mammalian erythrocytes, basophilic stippling in avian erythrocytes is considered evidence of degrading ribonucleoproteins and can be seen in regenerative anemia as a result of accelerated erythrocyte production or, rarely, because of lead toxicosis [1].

Hematologic abnormalities consistent with immune-mediated hemolytic anemia have been rarely reported in birds. Erythrocyte agglutination can be visualized microscopically in a stained blood smear or by performing a saline dispersion test, supporting cross-linking of erythrocytes by surface immunoglobulin. In addition, two clinical reports of avian patients that have disease resembling immune-mediated hemolytic anemia describe small round erythrocytes, potentially spherocytes, in blood smears from the patients [19].

Heinz bodies, aggregates of precipitating denatured hemoglobin, have been documented in avian erythrocytes. In birds, Heinz bodies are small, round to irregular, and often multiple inclusions that stain light blue with new methylene blue staining and can occur in the cytoplasm and the nucleus

[11]. They may also be seen as refractile inclusions in unstained blood smears and appear as more densely staining hemoglobin aggregates in Wright's-stained smears. Heinz bodies form as a result of oxidative damage to the hemoglobin molecule and cause increased rigidity of the erythrocyte membrane. Decreased deformability may lead to intravascular lysis of the erythrocyte or phagocytosis within the splenic microcirculation. Hemolytic anemia and Heinz bodies have been documented in marine birds exposed to petroleum products [11,20]. Geese fed green onions in one study infrequently developed erythrocyte Heinz bodies compatible with evidence implicating several thiosulfate compounds present in onions and onion products as causes of Heinz body hemolytic anemia in cats and other domestic animal species [21,22].

Clinical approach to avian anemia

Challenges faced by a clinician evaluating an avian patient that has anemia include recognizing clinically that anemia is present, determining the severity and chronicity of the anemia, determining the underlying cause, treating the underlying cause, and deciding whether treatment for the anemia itself is warranted. Clinical signs of anemia include weakness, lethargy, collapse, and respiratory signs. Physical examination findings that lead to a suspicion of anemia include pale oral or cloacal mucous membranes, decreased cutaneous ulnar vein size, poor peripheral arterial pulses, tachycardia, and a physiologic heart murmur. There may be obvious signs of blood loss, such as trauma, broken blood feathers, bruising, melena, or hematochezia. There may not be an obvious cause for the anemia, however, and additional diagnostics must be performed.

When anemia is suspected, a blood sample should be collected and the PCV and RBC morphology should be evaluated. In general, anemia in birds is defined as a PCV of less than 35% [7]. For many psittacines, however, normal PCV is greater than 45%; therefore reference ranges for individual species should be consulted [23]. The severity of the anemia should be assessed. A PCV of 25% to 35% indicates mild to moderate anemia, whereas a PCV of less than 20% is a severe anemia [24]. It is important to determine whether the anemia is regenerative or nonregenerative. As mentioned previously, a reticulocyte count is the best method for determining regeneration [10]. If this technique is not available, however, the degree of polychromasia can also be used to estimate regeneration. Because a small amount of polychromasia is normal in the absence of anemia, moderate (2+) or higher polychromasia would be expected with a regenerative anemia. Differentials for regenerative anemia include acute blood loss or hemolysis. Acute blood loss, such as is caused by trauma, gastrointestinal (GI) bleeding (eg, parasitism, GI ulceration, GI neoplasia), or coagulopathy (eg, rodenticides, erythremic myelosis syndrome, secondary to aflatoxicosis), is the most common cause of regenerative anemia in birds [5,25]. Hemolytic anemia in birds has also been reported. Causes of hemolytic anemia include hemic parasites, septicemia (ie, salmonellosis), toxins (eg, lead, zinc, petroleum products), and immune-mediated hemolytic anemia [5,11,19,26,27]. Additional diagnostic tests, such as a slide agglutination test, radiographs, liver aspirate, liver biopsy, splenic biopsy, and bone marrow aspirate, can be used to confirm hemolysis and to evaluate for an underlying cause [19,26]. The differential diagnoses for nonregenerative anemia include anemia of chronic disease (especially chlamydophilosis, mycobacteriosis, aspergillosis, West Nile virus, or neoplasia), toxicity (eg, lead toxicosis, aflatoxicosis), iron deficiency, hypothyroidism, and leukemia [1,5,28–30]. Additional diagnostics, such as infectious disease testing, toxicology, radiology, ultrasound, and bone marrow aspiration, may be required to diagnose the cause of a nonregenerative anemia. Bone marrow aspirates may be collected from the proximal tibiotarsus, sternum, or long bones that are not pneumatized. The proximal tibiotarsus is the most common site that is used. Birds should be anesthetized before collection of bone marrow because of pain and stress associated with the procedure. Details on the collection, preparation, and interpretation of bone marrow aspirates have been previously described [1,31].

Volume support and blood transfusions

Treatment of anemia in birds involves identifying the underlying cause, treating or removing the underlying cause, providing supportive care, and, in some cases, providing blood transfusions. Supportive care includes administration of crystalloid fluids, colloidal fluids, iron dextran, and vitamin B [24,32,33]. Oxyglobin (Biopure Corporation, Cambridge, Massachusetts) may also be used for support of anemic patients. Oxyglobin is a purified polymerized bovine hemoglobin product in lactated Ringer's solution. It is approved for use in dogs but has been successfully used in exotic species, including birds, when whole blood is not available for transfusion [33,34]. Oxyglobin is also useful in the treatment of hemorrhagic shock because it has a vasoconstrictive effect that can decrease the volume necessary for resuscitation [34]. Because Oxyglobin is a colloid, it should be used cautiously in birds that are normovolemic or hypervolemic [34].

Whether to administer a blood transfusion to an anemic bird depends on several variables. In general, transfusion is recommended for birds with a PCV of less than 20%. There are exceptions to this, however. For instance, birds with chronic anemia may acclimate to a lower PCV and fail to demonstrate clinical signs of anemia even with a PCV less than 20%. Blood transfusion is not indicated in these birds unless they are undergoing a major procedure, such as surgery. Transfusion is also contraindicated in some cases of acute blood loss. Pigeons have been demonstrated experimentally to survive acute blood loss of up to 70% of the blood volume [24]. Birds that are otherwise healthy can recover to a normal PCV in 3 to 6 days after acute blood loss [24,35]. Therefore, birds in good health that experience acute blood loss, such as from a broken blood feather, may only require fluid therapy, supportive care, and time to recover from the event. Another factor that is important in determining whether to perform a transfusion is the species of the donor and recipient birds. There is limited information available regarding blood groups in avian species. Chickens have been demonstrated to have at least 28 different blood group antigens, and blood groups have also been studied in other Galliformes and waterfowl [36,37]. There is no published information available about blood groups in psittacine species. It has been shown that birds do not have preformed antigens to blood groups, however; therefore, a single blood transfusion, even from a donor from a different species or genus (heterologous blood transfusion), may be safely administered [24,38–40]. After the initial transfusion, birds become sensitized to donor antigens; therefore, multiple transfusions carry the risk for fatal reactions [41]. RBCs from donors of the same species as the recipient (homologous blood transfusions) have been shown to survive significantly longer than RBCs from heterologous transfusions [38–40]. Although the RBCs provided by a heterologous transfusion can provide support in the short term, the added physiologic stress of hemolysis and removal of cellular breakdown products by the recipient may negate the benefits of the transfusion. Therefore, whenever possible, a homologous transfusion should be performed. In the absence of a donor of the same species, Oxyglobin may be a superior choice to a heterologous transfusion. The exception is birds with significant ongoing bleeding; in such a case, the transfusion may be lifesaving. A cross-match should be performed before administration of a blood transfusion if time and sample volume allow, and birds should be monitored for transfusion reactions, although transfusion reactions have not been reported in birds [34]. Blood transfusions and Oxyglobin may be administered by means of intravenous or intraosseous catheters [34,41]. Methods for collection, storage, and administration of blood have been previously described [34,37,41]. Blood must be collected fresh because none of the storage media currently available preserves avian blood without the development of dangerously high levels of potassium [42].

Polycythemia

Polycythemia, or an increase in the PCV and RBC count, is an uncommon finding in birds. Generally polycythemia in birds is defined as a PCV greater than 70% [1]. There are two main categories of polycythemia: absolute and relative. Relative polycythemia results from dehydration and a loss of plasma volume and can be corrected by rehydrating the bird and treating the cause of the dehydration. Absolute polycythemia can be further divided into two categories: primary polycythemia and secondary polycythemia. Primary polycythemia, or polycythemia vera, is a rare finding in birds but can occur [1]. This condition is caused by a myeloproliferative disorder that results in an increase in erythrocytosis. Diagnosis of polycythemia vera requires ruling out secondary causes of polycythemia. Secondary polycythemia occurs as a result of an increased need for tissue oxygenation or because of an increase in the production of erythropoietin. Examples of diseases that lead to secondary polycythemia include chronic pulmonary disease, adaptation to high altitude, cardiac disease, iron storage disease, rickets, or renal disease or neoplasia leading to increased production of erythropoietin [1,43]. Treatment of polycythemia involves treatment of the underlying cause and periodic phlebotomy.

Avian leukocytes and related disorders

Avian leukocytes can be divided into granulocytes, lymphocytes, and mononuclear cells. Granulocytes, named for their conspicuous cytoplasmic granules, include heterophils, eosinophils, and basophils.

Heterophils

Heterophils are the most common granulocyte involved in the acute inflammatory response in avian species. In Wright's-stained preparations of avian blood smears, mature heterophils are round cells with a lobed basophilic nucleus and prominent eosinophilic (orange red to red brown) needle-shaped granules (Fig. 4). There is variation among bird species in the shape of the cytoplasmic granules from oval to round. The cytoplasm of heterophils is generally colorless.

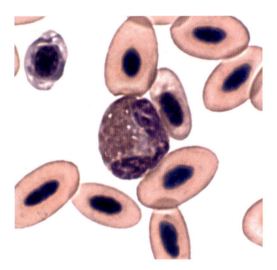

Fig. 4. Normal avian heterophil surrounded by erythrocytes. Note the lobed basophilic nucleus and the rod-shaped orange-brown eosinophilic cytoplasmic granules.

There are two common types of changes observed in heterophils during the course of disease processes in birds. One change is the presence of immature cells in the peripheral blood, representing recruitment of cells from the bone marrow in response to cytokines and other inflammatory mediators [1]. These immature cells have more basophilic cytoplasm than mature heterophils, have nonsegmented nuclei, and have granules that are immature. Band heterophils are similar to mature heterophils, except the nucleus is horseshoe shaped with parallel sides and lacks lobules. Often, the nucleus is obscured by the cytoplasmic granules. Metamyelocytes and myelocytes are less mature cells and are larger than band heterophils (Fig. 5). The nucleus of these cells is round to oval, and the cytoplasm is basophilic. Myelocytes and metamyelocytes have spiculate cytoplasmic granules; however, in myelocytes, the granules take up less than one half of the cytoplasm, whereas in metamyelocytes, the granules take up more than one half of the cytoplasm [1]. Band heterophils are identified in peripheral blood smears in the first 12 to 24 hours after an inflammatory event [44]. This left shift peaks at approximately 12 hours after the initial insult in chickens, with persistence of leukocytosis for 7 days [44]. The presence of immature cells in avian blood smears indicates acute inflammation. A degenerative left shift, in which the number of immature heterophils exceeds the number of mature heterophils, indicates an intense tissue demand for cells and carries a poor prognosis.

The other important change observed in avian heterophils during disease is toxic change. Toxic changes observed in avian heterophils are similar to those observed in mammalian neutrophils. Characteristics of toxicity

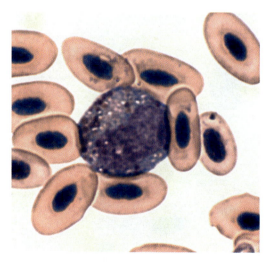

Fig. 5. Heterophil metamyelocyte demonstrates toxic change. The nucleus is oval, and the cytoplasm is basophilic. Many of the cytoplasmic granules are basophilic. The granules take up more than 50% of the cytoplasm, characterizing this cell as a metamyelocyte rather than a myelocyte.

include cell swelling, basophilic cytoplasm, vacuolation of the cytoplasm, changes in granules, such as basophilic staining or granules that coalesce into larger granules, and hypersegmentation and degeneration of the nucleus (see Fig. 5; Fig. 6) [44]. Degranulation may also occur, but caution should be used in interpreting degranulation in peripheral blood smears because this can be an artifact of smear preparation or staining [45]. Toxicity is generally reported on a scale of 1+ to 4+, with 4+ representing the most severe toxic changes. In addition, the proportion of heterophils exhibiting toxicity should be reported as a percentage or as few, moderate, or marked. The presence of toxic heterophils indicates an inflammatory response associated with severe systemic disease.

The avian heterophil generally corresponds to the mammalian neutrophil, although there are important distinctions. Avian heterophils perform phagocytosis, have bactericidal properties, and have roles in acute inflammation. Avian heterophils do not contain the enzyme myeloperoxidase, the main lysosomal enzyme present in mammalian neutrophils, which functions in phagolysosomal killing. Heterophil granules do contain bactericidal lysosomal and nonlysosomal enzymes that function in phagocytosis and destruction of bacterial organisms, however. Avian heterophils are involved in controlling bacterial, viral, and parasitic infections. One key difference between birds and mammals is the process of pus formation. In mammals, neutrophils accumulate, leading to liquefaction and abscess formation. This liquid pus can spread along tissue planes or can form exudates that are removed by way of clearance pathways such as the mucociliary apparatus [46]. In contrast, in birds, heterophils accumulate and are resolved by

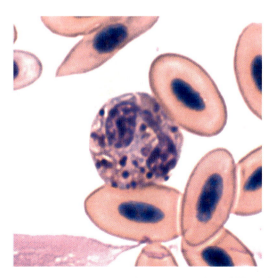

Fig. 6. Toxic change in a mature heterophil. The cytoplasm is basophilic, and cytoplasmic vacuolation is present. Several of the heterophilic granules are basophilic rather than eosinophilic.

means of inspissation of necrotic heterophils into a caseous mass rather than liquefaction. The necrotic heterophils are walled off by epithelioid macrophages and fibrous connective tissue to form heterophilic granulomas [46]. This process is advantageous, except when the caseous masses that are formed interfere with organ formation, such as in granulomas in the lungs or air sacs. In certain locations, these caseous masses could persist indefinitely. The exact mechanism of pus formation in birds has not been completely elucidated. Proposed mechanisms include variances in hydrolytic enzyme activity, such as the lack of myeloperoxidase in heterophils, or the lack of as yet to be identified proteases in birds [46].

Conditions that cause an increase in heterophils in the peripheral blood include infection (eg, bacterial, fungal, viral, parasitic), inflammation, stress, certain toxicities, trauma, and leukemia [47–49]. Common infectious agents that lead to heterophilia include *Mycobacterium* spp, *Chlamydophila psittaci*, and *Aspergillus* spp. Heterophilia associated with infections with these organisms is also commonly accompanied by monocytosis. Chickens acutely or chronically infected with *Mycoplasma* spp also developed heterophilia and monocytosis [50]. It has been demonstrated that heterophils are the predominant component of exudates in birds, although lymphocytes and basophils may also be present early in inflammation [46]. Heterophilia with toxic change is indicative of severe systemic illness, such as septicemia, chlamydophilosis, fungal infection, or viremia. The development of toxic change may indicate lack of control of an infectious process and often carries a poor prognosis, especially with 3 to 4+ toxic change [1].

Certain toxins can lead to heterophilia in birds. For example, heterophilia was observed in a swan with organophosphate toxicity [51]. In addition, heterophilia has been observed in cases of zinc toxicosis, presumably as a result of GI inflammation, stress, and decreased resistance to pathogens [1].

A stress response similar to that seen in mammals has been reported in birds. For example, macaws may demonstrate marked leukocytosis with heterophilia as a result of transport and handling. The administration of corticosteroids results in an increase in circulating heterophils and lymphopenia in chickens [46]. In chickens, the heterophil-to-lymphocyte (H/L) ratio is a useful tool for monitoring stress responses [52].

A decrease in heterophil numbers can be seen with increased use of cells or decreased production. Utilization of mature cells and a resultant left shift can be seen 12 to 24 hours after the initiation of acute inflammation [44]. Overwhelming infection, such as septicemia, can lead to a degenerative left shift, which indicates bone marrow depletion. Psittacine circovirus can lead to leukopenia with pancytopenia in African gray parrots [53].

Eosinophils

Eosinophils are round granulocytes that are similar in size to avian heterophils. The eosinophil nucleus is lobed and basophilic, whereas the cytoplasm stains clear blue with Wright's stain (Fig. 7). The granules are brightly eosinophilic and tend to be round as opposed to the needle-shaped granules of heterophils. The cytoplasmic granules of avian eosinophils lack the central refractile body that is observed in avian heterophils [1]. Variation among species and staining artifact can lead to granules that are colorless or blue. Comparison with other cells on the slide must be made to identify these cells as eosinophils.

The granules of avian eosinophils are similar to mammalian counterparts, containing lysozymes, peroxidase, and high concentrations of arginine [1,54]. The exact function of avian eosinophils is unclear, however [54]. In mammals, eosinophils are modulators of immediate hypersensitivity and suppress parasitic infections. Some studies have shown a limited association between eosinophils and nematode infection in grouse and other fowl [55]. Parasite antigens do not generally induce eosinophilia in birds, however. Other studies have shown eosinophilia with generalized inflammation in birds. It is possible that avian eosinophils play a role in delayed hypersensitivity, but they have not been shown to be related to anaphylaxis or other acute hypersensitivity reactions [54]. The authors have also observed severe eosinophilia in cases of poxvirus infection in red-tailed hawks, although the mechanism of this response is unknown (Mitchell, unpublished data, 2007).

Basophils

Avian basophils are slightly smaller than heterophils and have a colorless cytoplasm. They contain intensely basophilic granules, although the granules may dissolve, coalesce, or appear abnormal when stained with

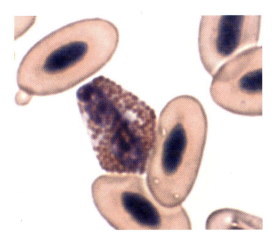

Fig. 7. Avian eosinophil. The nucleus is basophilic and lobed. The cytoplasmic granules are brightly eosinophilic and rounded.

alcohol-based stains, such as Wright's stain (Fig. 8). The nucleus of baso-phils, often obscured by the granules, is round to oval and nonlobed. Baso-phils are much more common in avian peripheral blood smears than in mammalian blood smears.

The function of avian basophils is unknown. Basophils seem to be in-volved in the initial phases of acute inflammation, but this does not always result in peripheral basophilia [54]. The granules of avian basophils contain histamine, as in mammals [1]. Therefore, it is suggested that they function in acute inflammatory and type IV hypersensitivity reactions, similar to mam-malian basophils and mast cells.

Lymphocytes

Avian lymphocytes are similar in morphology to mammalian lympho-cytes. They are round cells with centrally positioned or slightly eccentric nuclei (Fig. 9). The chromatin in the nucleus is densely aggregated, and there is a high nuclear-to-cytoplasmic (N/C) ratio. The cytoplasm is basophilic and homogeneous, with no vacuolation. Generally, there are no granules in lymphocytes, although, occasionally, rare azurophilic granules may be present. There is frequently variation in size of avian lymphocytes, and they can be difficult to distinguish from other cells. Small lymphocytes often resemble thrombocytes. Thrombocytes can be distinguished by the presence of clear colorless cytoplasm, vacuolation, and few azurophilic granules (see Fig. 9). Large lymphocytes may be difficult to distinguish from monocytes. Monocytes differ from lymphocytes by their large size, more abundant cyto-plasmic volume, and less densely clumped chromatin. Plasma cells, which are large B lymphocytes, are sometimes observed in avian blood smears.

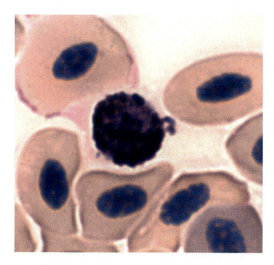

Fig. 8. Avian basophil. The granules are densely basophilic and obscure the nucleus.

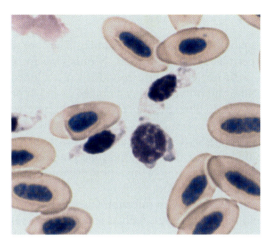

Fig. 9. Avian lymphocyte and two thrombocytes. The lymphocyte is larger with a round nucleus and a basophilic cytoplasm that lacks vacuoles. The thrombocytes have a clear to pale gray vacuolated cytoplasm.

These cells are large with eccentrically located nuclei, an intensely basophilic cytoplasm, and a distinct Golgi zone.

Reactive lymphocytes are small to medium sized with densely clumped chromatin and intensely basophilic cytoplasm. Nucleoli are usually absent, and a pale Golgi zone and vacuolation may be present. Reactive lymphocytes can be seen in small numbers in peripheral blood smears of healthy birds. Increased numbers of reactive lymphocytes suggest that antigenic stimulation is occurring. Increased numbers of reactive lymphocytes are commonly observed in birds that have infectious diseases. Blast-transformed lymphocytes may also occasionally be observed in avian blood smears. These are large lymphocytes with smooth dispersed chromatin and nucleoli often present. There is abundant blue cytoplasm, and there is often a prominent Golgi zone. These cells can be neoplastic, indicating lymphoid leukemia or a leukemic phase of lymphoma, but can also be seen as a result of immunologic stimulation.

Lymphocytosis usually occurs as a result of antigenic stimulation. This can occur in psittacine birds with viral disease, such as herpesvirus or psittacine circovirus [45]. This result is inconsistent, however, and the same viral diseases may instead result in heterophilia or leukopenia [45,53]. Lymphocytosis may be seen in birds with lymphoid leukemia. Anemia and thrombocytopenia may also be present in birds with lymphocytic leukemia [56]. Lymphocytic leukemias are rare in birds in comparison to lymphosarcoma [28]. Certain species of birds are normally lymphocytic, with lymphocytes representing up to 70% of leukocytes. Examples of lymphocytic species include Amazon parrots and canaries. Lymphopenia may be seen as a result of excess endogenous or exogenous corticosteroids [46].

Monocytes

Avian and mammalian monocytes are similar. They are the largest leukocyte in normal peripheral blood smears. Monocytes are round or amor-
phous in shape, with nuclei that are round, oval, or lobed (Fig. 10). The
chromatin is lacelike and not as densely clumped as in lymphocytes. The cytoplasm of monocytes is blue gray and contains discrete vacuoles and fine
eosinophilic granules.

Monocytes have phagocytic activity and transform into macrophages after they migrate into tissues. Their cytoplasmic granules contain lysozymes
that are involved in destruction of invading organisms and chemicals involved in mediating inflammation.

Monocytosis is often seen with infectious or inflammatory disease, especially with granulomatous diseases, such as aspergillosis or mycobacteriosis.
Birds with *Chlamydophila psittaci* infections also often develop monocytosis
because of the production of chemotactic agents that attract monocytes [5].
Other bacterial granulomas or massive tissue necrosis may also induce
monocytosis [5]. Although monocytosis is common with chronic inflammation, acute infections, such as *Mycoplasma* spp infections, may lead to
monocytosis in addition to heterophilia and lymphopenia [50]. Monocytosis
may also be observed in birds fed a zinc-deficient diet [57].

Thrombocytes

Thrombocytes are small oval- to rectangular-shaped cells with a round
nucleus that contains densely clumped purple-red chromatin (see Fig. 9)
[1]. There is a high N/C ratio, and the nucleus is more rounded than the nucleus of erythrocytes. Distinguishing thrombocytes from small lymphocytes

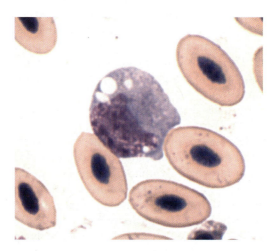

Fig. 10. Avian monocyte. Note the oval slightly lobed nucleus with loosely clumped chromatin,
the blue-gray cytoplasm, and the vacuolation of the cytoplasm.

can be challenging. The cytoplasm of thrombocytes is colorless to pale gray blue and may be reticulated, may contain large vacuoles, or may contain eosinophilic granules [1]. Avian thrombocytes are derived from stem cell precursors rather than from megakaryocytes as in mammals. Similar to platelets in mammals, thrombocytes function in hemostasis and produce thromboplastin. Avian thrombocytes are also phagocytic and have a minor role in removing foreign materials from the blood [58]. The importance of thrombocytes in fighting infection in avian species is unknown. Thrombocyte counts are not generally performed in avian hematology because clumping is frequent. Therefore, thrombocytes are generally described as decreased, adequate, or increased.

Thrombocytopenia can be seen with increased destruction or use, such as septicemia or possibly disseminated intravascular coagulation (DIC). Thrombocytopenia can be seen as a component of pancytopenia in some viral diseases, such as psittacine circovirus or polyomavirus infections [59]. It has also been reported in cases of lymphoid leukemia [56]. Thrombocytosis and an increase in the size of thrombocytes may be seen with chronic inflammation in birds [60].

Hemic parasites

Hemic parasites most commonly found in avian blood smears include *Plasmodium*, *Hemoproteus*, and *Leukocytozoon*. *Plasmodium* spp organisms can be pathogenic, causing avian malaria in susceptible birds, including canaries, ducks, raptors, penguins, and domestic poultry. Clinical and hematologic signs of disease include anorexia, hemolytic anemia, leukocytosis and lymphocytosis, and death. Intraerythrocytic gametocytes can be found in blood smears. Gametocytes contain refractile iron pigment, vary from round to elongate in shape, and cause variable displacement of the erythrocyte nucleus (Fig. 11). Schizonts composed of immature or mature merozoites may be found in erythrocytes, and gametocytes and schizonts can be seen in other hemic cells [7]. Small ring-like trophozoites can also be seen in erythrocytes. Mosquitos are intermediate hosts for *Plasmodium*.

Hemoproteus gametocytes also contain refractile iron pigment and are found in erythrocytes (Fig. 12). *Hemoproteus* differs from *Plasmodium* in that gametocytes often encircle more than half of the erythrocyte nucleus without displacing the nucleus and are not found in other hemic cells. Extracellular macrogametes and microgametes may be seen as erythrocytes lyse with sample aging. *Hemoproteus* is generally of low pathogenicity but may cause hemolytic anemia in pigeons, quail, and ill birds in general. A decrease in the percentage of infected erythrocytes is considered to reflect improved immune status in raptors and other birds [7]. Hippoboscid flies and midges are intermediate hosts of *Hemoproteus*.

Leukocytozoon infection is common in wild birds and is also considered to be of low pathogenicity, although susceptible birds, such as turkeys

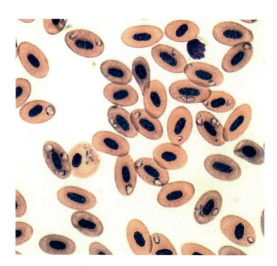

Fig. 11. Avian blood smear with *Plasmodium* parasites within erythrocytes. Several life stages, including gametocytes and trophozoites, can be seen within individual erythrocytes. Refractile iron pigment can be seen in several organisms.

and young waterfowl, may develop hemolytic anemia. Gametocytes can be found in hemic cells, in which they markedly distort the cell and displace the nucleus (Fig. 13). It is debated whether leukocytes or erythrocytes are the hemic cell type infected. It is currently believed that both cell types are infected by *Leukocytozoon* gametocytes, with erythrocytes more commonly

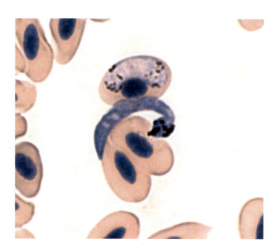

Fig. 12. *Hemoproteus* hemic parasites. The erythrocyte at the top of the image contains a gametocyte with refractile iron pigment. The gametocyte of *Hemoproteus* can be identified by the fact that it encircles more than half of the erythrocyte nucleus without displacing the nucleus. In the center of the image is an extracellular *Hemoproteus* gamete. These occur in blood films because of lysis of the erythrocytes as the sample ages.

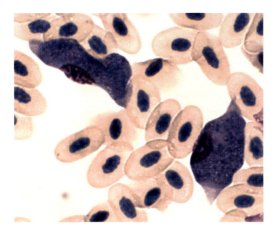

Fig. 13. Avian blood smear with *Leukocytozoon* hemic parasites. Large deeply basophilic macrogametocytes are observed distorting the shape of the cells.

affected [61]. Gametocytes are often elongated to spindloid but can also be rounded depending on the species of organism. Macrogametes are dark blue with a compact dark nucleus, whereas microgametocytes are pale blue with a diffuse pink nucleus [61]. Blackflies are the primary intermediate host of *Leukocytozoon*.

Summary

Avian hematology is an essential diagnostic tool in avian practice that aids in diagnosis of disease processes. There are many similarities between avian hematology and mammalian hematology that can be useful to the practitioner in evaluating avian blood smears. There are also important differences that must be taken into account, however, such as the presence of nucleated RBCs, the presence of heterophils as opposed to neutrophils, and differences in the function of cells. There is still a large amount to be learned about the functions of avian blood cells, and research in this field is ongoing. It is hoped that this overview of avian hematology and associated changes observed during disease aids the practitioner in evaluating blood smears, interpreting changes observed in avian blood cells, developing differential lists, and successfully treating avian patients.

References

[1] Campbell TW, Ellis CK. Hematology of birds. In: Campbell TW, Ellis CK, editors. Avian and exotic animal hematology and cytology. 3rd edition. Ames (IA): Blackwell Publishing Professional; 2007. p. 3–50.

[2] Fudge AM. Avian blood sampling and artifact considerations. In: Fudge AM, editor. Laboratory medicine: avian and exotic pets. Philadelphia: Saunders; 2000. p. 1–8.

[3] Walberg J. White blood cell counting techniques in birds. Seminars in Avian and Exotic Pet Medicine 2001;10(2):72–6.

[4] Kass L, Harrison GJ, Lindheimer C. A new stain for identification of avian leukocytes. Biotech Histochem 2002;77(4):201–6.

[5] Campbell T. Hematology. In: Ritchie BW, Harrison GJ, Harrison LR, editors. Avian medicine: principles and application. Lake Worth (FL): Wingers Publishing; 1994. p. 176–98.

[6] Herbert R, Nanney J, Spano JS, et al. Erythrocyte distribution in ducks. Am J Vet Res 1989; 50(6):958–60.

[7] Thrall MA. Hematology of birds. In: Thrall MA, Baker DC, Campbell TW, et al, editors. Veterinary hematology and clinical chemistry. Baltimore (MD): Lippincott, Williams and Wilkins; 2004. p. 225–58.

[8] Sturkie PD, Griminger P. Body fluids: blood. In: Sturkie P, editor. Avian physiology. 4th edition. New York: Springer-Verlag; 1986. p. 102–29.

[9] Natt MP, Herrick CA. A new blood diluent for counting erythrocytes and leucocytes of the chicken. Poult Sci 1952;31:735–8.

[10] Johns JL, Shooshtari MP, Christopher MM. Development of a technique for quantification of avian reticulocytes. Am J Vet Res, in press.

[11] Leighton FA. Morphological lesions in red blood cells from herring gulls and Atlantic puffins ingesting Prudhoe Bay crude oil. Vet Pathol 1985;22(4):393–402.

[12] Gurd MR. The use of grain-fed pigeons in the biological assay of liver preparations. Q J Pharm Pharmacol 1935;8:39–53.

[13] Lucas AM, Jamroz C. Atlas of avian hematology. Washington, DC: USDA; 1961.

[14] Christopher MM, Shooshtari MP, Levengood JM. Assessment of erythrocyte morphologic abnormalities in mallards with experimentally induced zinc toxicosis. Am J Vet Res 2004; 65(4):440–6.

[15] Storey ML, Greger JL. Iron, zinc and copper interactions: chronic versus acute responses of rats. J Nutr 1987;117:1434–42.

[16] Pimental JL, Greger JL, Cook MF, et al. Iron metabolism in chicks fed various levels of zinc and copper. J Nutr Biochem 1992;13:140–5.

[17] Romagnano A, Grindem CB, Degernes LA, et al. Treatment of a hyacinth macaw with zinc toxicity. J Avian Med Surg 1995;9:185–9.

[18] Fudge AM. Disorders of avian erythrocytes. In: Fudge AM, editor. Laboratory medicine: avian and exotic pets. Philadelphia: Saunders; 2000. p. 28–34.

[19] Johnston MS, Son TT, Rosenthal KL. Immune-mediated hemolytic anemia in an eclectus parrot. J Am Vet Med Assoc 2007;230(7):1028–31.

[20] Troisi G, Borjesson L, Bexton S. Biomarkers of polycyclic aromatic hydrocarbon (PAH)-associated hemolytic anemia in oiled wildlife. Environ Res 2007;105(3):324–9.

[21] Robertson JE, Christopher MM, Rogers QR. Heinz body formation in cats fed baby food containing onion powder. J Am Vet Med Assoc 1998;212:1260–6.

[22] Crespo R, Chin RP. Effect of feeding green onions (Allium ascalonicum) to white Chinese geese (Threskiornis spinicollis). J Vet Diagn Invest 2004;16(4):321–5.

[23] Polo FJ, Peinado VI, Viscor G, et al. Hematologic and plasma chemistry values in captive psittacine birds. Avian Dis 1998;42(3):523–35.

[24] Bos JH, Todd B, Tell LA, et al. Treatment of anemic birds with iron dextran therapy: homologous and heterologous blood transfusions. In: Proceedings of the Association of Avian Veterinarians. Phoenix (AZ): September 10–15, 1990. p. 221–5.

[25] Goodman GJ. Metabolic disorders. In: Rosskopf WJ, Woerpel RW, editors. Diseases of cage and aviary birds. Baltimore (MD): Williams & Wilkins; 1996. p. 470–9.

[26] Jones JS, Thomas JS, Bahr A, et al. Presumed immune-mediated hemolytic anemia in a blue-crowned conure (Aratinga acuticaudata). J Avian Med Surg 2002;16(3):223–9.

[27] Ochiai K, Jin K, Goryo M, et al. Pathomorphologic findings of lead poisoning in white-fronted geese (Anser albifrons). Vet Pathol 1993;30(6):522–8.

[28] Newell S, McMillan M, Moore F. Diagnosis and treatment of lymphocytic leukemia and malignant lymphoma in a Pekin duck (Anas platyrhynchos domesticus). Journal of the Association of Avian Veterinarians 1991;5(2):83–6.

[29] Tell LA, Woods L, Cromie RL. Mycobacteriosis in birds. Rev Sci Tech 2001;20(1):180–203.

[30] Joyner PH, Kelly S, Shreve AA, et al. West Nile virus in raptors from Virginia during 2003: clinical, diagnostic, and epidemiologic findings. J Wildl Dis 2006;42(2):335–44.

[31] Murray MJ. Diagnostic techniques in avian medicine. Sem Av Exotic Pet 1997;6(2):48–54.

[32] Rupley AE. Emergency procedures: recovering from disaster [abstract 6000]. In: Proceedings of the Association of Avian Veterinarians. Reno (NV): September 10–12, 1997. p. 249–57.

[33] Lichtenberger M, Rosenthal K, Brue R, et al. Administration of oxyglobin and 6% hetastarch after acute blood loss in psittacine birds [abstract 1040]. In: Proceedings of the Association of Avian Veterinarians. Orlando (FL): August 22–24, 2001. p. 15–8.

[34] Lichtenberger M. Transfusion medicine in exotic pets. Clin Tech Small Anim Pract 2004; 19(2):88–95.

[35] Ploucha JM, Scott JB, Ringer RK. Vascular and hematologic effects of hemorrhage in the chicken. Am J Physiol 1981;240(1):H9–17.

[36] Gilmour DG. Blood groups. In: Freeman BM, editor. Physiology and biochemistry of the domestic fowl, vol. 5. New York: Academic Press; 1984. p. 263–76.

[37] Morrisey JK. Transfusion medicine in birds (VET-598). In: Proceedings of the Western Veterinary Conference. Las Vegas (NV): February 8–12, 2004.

[38] Sandmeier P, Stauber EH, Wardrop KJ, et al. Survival of pigeon red blood cells after transfusion into selected raptors. J Am Vet Med Assoc 1994;204(3):427–9.

[39] Degernes LA, Crosier ML, Harrison LD, et al. Autologous, homologous, and heterologous red blood cell transfusions in cockatiels (Nymphicus hollandicus). J Avian Med Surg 1999; 13(1):2–9.

[40] Degernes LA, Harrison LD, Smith DW, et al. Autologous, homologous, and heterologous red blood cell transfusions in conures of the genus Aratinga. J Avian Med Surg 1999;13(1):10–4.

[41] Hoefer HL. Transfusions in exotic species. Probl Vet Med 1992;4(4):625–35.

[42] Morrisey JK, Giger U. Comparison of three media for the storage of avian whole blood [abstract 6040]. In: Proceedings of the Association of Avian Veterinarians. Reno (NV): September 10–12, 1997. p. 279–80.

[43] Samour J. Diagnostic value of hematology. In: Harrison GJ, Lightfoot TL, editors. Clinical avian medicine, vol. 2Palm Beach (FL): Spix Publishing; 2006. p. 587–610.

[44] Latimer KS, Tang KN, Goodwin MA, et al. Leukocyte changes associated with acute inflammation in chickens. Avian Dis 1988;32(4):760–72.

[45] Fudge AM, Joseph V. Disorders of avian leukocytes. In: Fudge AM, editor. Laboratory medicine: avian and exotic pets. Philadelphia: Saunders; 2000. p. 19–27.

[46] Harmon BG. Avian heterophils in inflammation and disease resistance. Poult Sci 1998;77(7): 972–7.

[47] Bienzle D, Smith DA. Heterophilic leucocytosis and granulocyte hyperplasia associated with infection in a cockatoo. Comparative Haematology International 1999;9(4):193–7.

[48] Andreasen JR Jr, Andreasen CB, Anwer M, et al. Heterophil chemotaxis in chickens with natural Staphylococcal infections. Avian Dis 1993;37(2):284–9.

[49] Gildersleeve RP, Satterlee DG, Scott TR, et al. Hematology of Japanese quail selected for high or low serum corticosterone responses to complex stressors. Comp Biochem Physiol A 1987;86(3):569–73.

[50] Branton SL, May JD, Lott BD, et al. Various blood parameters in commercial hens acutely and chronically infected with Mycoplasma gallisepticum and Mycoplasma synoviae. Avian Dis 1997;41(3):540–7.

[51] Heatley J, Jowett P. What is your diagnosis? J Avian Med Surg 2000;14(4):283–4.

[52] Post J, Rebel J, ter Huurne A. Automated blood cell count: a sensitive and reliable method to study corticosterone-related stress in broilers. Poult Sci 2003;82(4):591–5.

[53] Schoemaker NJ, Dorrestein GM, Latimer KS, et al. Severe leukopenia and liver necrosis in young African grey parrots (Psittacus erithacus erithacus) infected with psittacine circovirus. Avian Dis 2000;44(2):470–8.

[54] Montali RJ. Comparative pathology of inflammation in the higher vertebrates (reptiles, birds and mammals). J Comp Pathol 1988;99(1):1–26.

[55] Maxwell M, Burns R. Blood eosinophilia in adult bantams naturally infected with Trichostrongylus tenuis. Res Vet Sci 1985;39(1):122–3.

[56] Latimer KS. Oncology. In: Ritchie BW, Harrison GJ, Harrison LR, editors. Avian medicine: principles and application. Lake Worth (FL): Wingers Publishing; 1994. p. 640–72.

[57] Wight PAL, Dewar WA, Mackenzie GM. Monocytosis in experimental zinc deficiency of domestic birds. Avian Pathol 1980;9(1):61–6.

[58] Grecchi R, Saliba AM, Mariano M. Morphological changes, surface receptors and phagocytic potential of fowl mono-nuclear phagocytes and thrombocytes in vivo and in vitro. J Pathol 1980;130(1):23–31.

[59] Fudge AM. Avian clinical pathology—hematology and chemistry. In: Altman RB, Clubb SL, Dorrestein GM, et al, editors. Avian medicine and surgery. Philadelphia: WB Saunders; 1997. p. 142–57.

[60] D'Aloia M-A, Samour J, Howlett J, et al. Haemopathologic responses to chronic inflammation in the houbara bustard (Chlamydotis undulata macqueenii). Comparative Haematology International 1994;4(4):203–6.

[61] Remple J. Intracellular hematozoa of raptors: a review and update. J Avian Med Surg 2004; 18(2):75–88.

ELSEVIER
SAUNDERS

Vet Clin Exot Anim 11 (2008) 523–533

VETERINARY
CLINICS
Exotic Animal Practice

Clinical Hematology of Rodent Species

Anthony A. Pilny, DVM, DABVP–Avian

*Avian and Exotic Pet Medicine, Animal Specialty Center, 9 Odell Plaza, Yonkers,
NY 10701, USA*

Popular pets in the order classified as rodents represent a diverse group of animals, including rats, hamsters, gerbils, prairie dogs, chinchillas, and guinea pigs. As standards of veterinary care are constantly rising for more commonly owned companion pets such as dogs, cats, and horses, rodent owners are also expecting higher levels of medicine and surgery than ever before. Medications and supportive care alone are not enough, and thorough diagnostic evaluation is mandated when pet rodents are ill or require anesthetic procedures. Because rodents are used in biomedical research, clinically useful information trickles down from the laboratory animal community, providing vital medical knowledge for veterinarians.

This article does not rehash basic information on restraint and blood collection in rodents but reviews concepts of clinical hematology and imparts information not widely available to clinical veterinarians who treat these much-valued pets. Readers are referred to specific textbooks and previously published issues of *Veterinary Clinics of North America: Exotic Animal Practice* for basic information on restraint and normal hematologic values.

Basic concepts

Because of the small size of rodents, the amount of blood that can be safely collected is essential to understand and estimate. As a general rule, the maximum that should be collected from a healthy patient is 1% of the body weight in kilograms. (eg, a 120 g hamster could tolerate collection of 1.2 mL of blood.) Possible continued loss through hematoma formation or bleeding is also important to consider, because this blood is unavailable to the circulatory system. Therefore, collecting half of the safe amount is best, assuming the sample will be appropriate for testing.

E-mail address: apilny@animalspecialtycenter.com

1094-9194/08/$ - see front matter © 2008 Elsevier Inc. All rights reserved.
doi:10.1016/j.cvex.2008.04.001

To maximize diagnostic value of a small blood sample, blood should be collected into a microtainer tube with the appropriate anticoagulant, preferably lithium heparin (Fig. 1). Wiedmeyer and colleagues [1] found that the quality of blood smears and complete blood cell (CBC) count results from the lithium heparin tube were comparable to those from an EDTA tube. Plasma is preferable to serum because the volume yield of plasma is greater than that of serum for a given amount of blood when whole blood cannot be used. Special centrifuges are available to spin microtubes rapidly (Fig. 2).

A CBC count can be obtained from a good quality blood smear on microscope slides and a capillary tube rather than an EDTA tube. Also, capillary tubes can be filled with only a small amount of blood and the hematocrit estimated by aligning the top of the plasma to the 50% line and doubling the end result. Also, microhematocrit tubes with smaller diameters exist that are approximately half the size of a standard tube and use less blood with the same result (Fig. 3).

Lastly, the needle should always be removed and blood transferred directly into the tube after blood collection to minimize the possibility of hemolysis from using small gauge needles. The author uses BD brand 3/10 cc insulin syringes with removable needles for most blood collection (Fig. 4).

Veterinarians must understand that blood samples are often difficult to obtain from small rodents when discussing a diagnostic plan with owners. Many animals lack large enough superficial vessels and the deeper vessels may be covered with fat. In many cases, anesthesia is necessary to safely collect an appropriate sample. Several collection sites are used to obtain blood from rodents (Table 1).

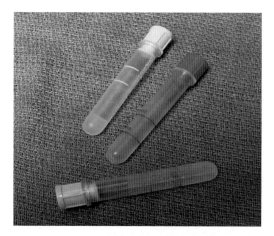

Fig. 1. Microtainer brand blood collection tubes appropriate for small samples. Lithium heparinized tubes are available with and without gel separator.

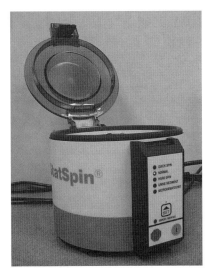

Fig. 2. Statspin centrifuge is designed to spin microhematocrit and microtainer tubes quietly and efficiently.

Techniques

Chinchilla, guinea pig, prairie dog

Sternal positioning, with the head and neck extended upward and forward, is best for performing jugular venipuncture of the chinchilla, guinea pig, and prairie dog, similar to a cat. Extending the neck forward is extremely important, because even slight caudal positioning can restrict respiration in these species. In chinchillas, the jugular vein is very superficial and the skin is thin. In guinea pigs, the jugular vein is located less superficially, the skin is thicker, and the vein is usually not visible or palpable.

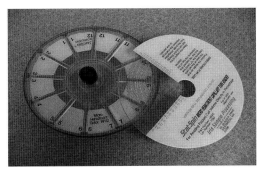

Fig. 3. Centrifuge adaptor for half size microhematocrit tubes. Less blood is required to obtain a patients hematocrit.

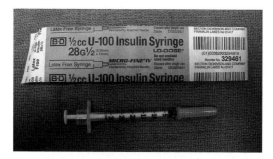

Fig. 4. BD U-100 insulin syringes are ideal for blood collection since needles are removable.

Prairie dogs are most challenging, with deeply located jugular veins surrounded by muscle and fat, and the entire cervical region is very short.

For cranial vena cava blood collection, the patient should be in dorsal recumbency with the front legs pulled caudally and apart. A small palpable divot is present in the junction formed between the point of the manubrium, the point of the sternum, and the first rib. A needle should be inserted at a 30° to 45° angle to the body, aiming toward the opposite back leg or kidney region. The angle may need to be varied slightly. Some patients should be sedated at the clinician's discretion before vena cava blood collection is attempted. The author masks down almost all patients with isoflurane or sevoflurane to facilitate collection. Venipuncture of the vena cava in guinea pigs has been reported to confer an increased risk for traumatic bleeding into the thoracic cavity or pericardial sac [2].

Peripheral vasculature, such as lateral saphenous veins, will yield small volumes of blood more appropriate for measuring packed cell volume, blood glucose, or tests requiring small volumes [3]. The author found that saphenous venipuncture is a fast, reliable method for blood collection in a range of species, and the position of the vein helps ensure that venipuncture is accurate, allowing for observation of any postcollection hemorrhage. It also eliminates the need for anesthesia when performed properly.

Table 1
Venipuncture sites in pet rodents

	Tail vein	Jugular vein	Lateral saphenous vein	Cranial vena cava	Femoral vein
Mice	X				
Rat	X	X	X		X
Hamster		X			X
Gerbil		X			
Prairie dog		X			
Chinchilla		X	X	X	X
Guinea Pig		X	X	X	X

Rats, hamsters, gerbils

General sedation is almost always required for blood collection of smaller rodents. Cranial vena cava blood collection may present more risk than larger rodents. A level of skill is required to access peripheral sites that are not always reliable for large volumes (Fig. 5). Lateral tail veins are easily accessed in rats, mice, and gerbils but are not recommended in gerbils as the tail is easily degloved.

Ventral tail artery venipuncture is usually performed in rats. In dorsal recumbency, the tail is approached at the ventral aspect, usually in the distal two thirds of the tail. A 27-gauge needle is inserted at the midline at approximately a 30° angle until the hub fills with blood with gentle suction. Blood will flow freely from this site into the needle and can be collected directly into tubes if preferred. Vasodilatation through warming can facilitate tail phlebotomy, and overuse of alcohol may make collection more difficult.

Orbital sinus and cardiac puncture are not considered humane methods of blood collection for pet rodents.

Hematologic features of rats and mice

The blood volume of the rat is reported as being between 5.0 and 7.1 mL per 100 g of body weight and approximately 5.5 mL/kg of blood can be withdrawn safely during a single collection. The mean total blood volume in mice has been calculated to be 5.85 mL per 100 g of body weight, and the mean plasma volume to be 3.15 mL per 100 g. Total blood volume in mice is 5.4% to 8.2% of body weight (average, 6.6%).

Hematologic parameters of mice and rats are influenced by several factors, such as collection site, age, gender, method of restraint, anesthesia, and level of stress. A circadian rhythm affects peripheral leukocyte concentration, with an increase during the light phase and decrease during the dark phase. In rats, blood collection through cardiopuncture is often inaccurate

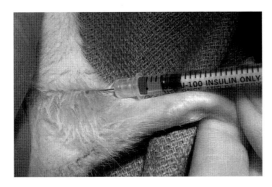

Fig. 5. Blood collection in the rat from the femoral vein. Samples up to 0.3 mL can be safely and quickly obtained from this site.

and often yields lower leukocyte and erythrocyte counts, hemoglobin concentration, and hematocrit percentages compared with samples from the tail. Stressed mice (eg, from transportation or handling) often show lowered total leukocyte concentrations. These factors are important when using and establishing reference ranges for these species, because collection method, environmental factors, and restraint may affect hematologic results.

The erythrocyte half-life in small rodents is from 45 to 67 days, which is shorter than for larger mammals. Polychromasia is a common finding on blood smears and adults normally have on average 2% to 7% reticulocytosis. Red blood cell concentrations are generally lower in females when compared with males.

Howell-Jolly bodies are found in low numbers of red cells of normal mice and rats. Rouleaux formation is uncommon, even in rats and mice with inflammatory disease. Granulocytes of mice and rats often have nuclei without distinct lobes and nuclei typically have a horseshoe or ring shape that develops from a hole in the nucleus during maturation. Segmentation occurs as the ring breaks and begins to form constrictions.

Neutrophils typically have a colorless cytoplasm but can contain few red granules and thus stain pink with Romanowsky stains. Eosinophils are larger than neutrophils and have a U-shaped or ring-shaped nucleus, basophilic cytoplasm, and numerous round cytoplasmic granules sometimes arranged in clumps. Basophils contain numerous basophilic granules and are present in small numbers in rats and mice. Basophils should be differentiated from circulating mast cells in peripheral blood. Lymphocyte size ranges from that of erythrocytes to that of neutrophils, with a light-blue staining cytoplasm and azurophilic cytoplasmic granules sometimes seen in large lymphocytes.

The leukocyte concentrations of rats and mice show diurnal variation and can vary among strains. An age-dependent variation exists in the neutrophil:lymphocyte ratio, with the neutrophil concentration increasing and lymphocyte concentration decreasing with age. Excitement and stress associated with blood collection in rats can alter white blood cell counts, causing an immediate leukocytosis and increase in circulating lymphocytes up to 12%. Ovariohysterectomy in rats results in an increase in the number and percentage of circulating T and B lymphocytes. Platelet counts tend to be higher in rats and mice compared with larger mammals, with counts greater than 1×10^6 cells/μL commonly found in healthy animals.

Hematologic features of guinea pigs

The blood volume of the adult guinea pig is approximately 69 to 75 mL per kilogram of body weight, and approximately 8% to 10% of the blood volume can be withdrawn safely in a single collection [4]. Guinea pigs have larger erythrocytes compared with other rodents, and polychromasia and macrocytosis are characteristic of regenerative anemias.

The neutrophils of guinea pigs contain eosinophilic-staining granules that are sometimes called *heterophils* and have the same function as in other mammals. The granules in eosinophils are larger than those in neutrophils and are often round to rod-shaped when compared. The granules of basophils are purple to black-staining.

Occasional Foa-Kurloff cells (KC cells), unique to guinea pigs, may be observed in circulation, accounting for up to 4% of the differential leukocyte count. These specialized mononuclear leukocytes contain an intracytoplasmic inclusion body consisting of a mucopolysaccharide and are called *Kurloff's Bodies* (Fig. 6). Males and females show no significant difference in numbers of observed KC cells after 2 to 3 months of age. Kurloff's bodies are highest in females during pregnancy and may help create a barrier between the developing fetus and the mother [4].

Hematologic features of mongolian gerbils

An erythrocytic macrocytosis, panleukocytosis, and erythrocyte counts lower than in adults has been observed in neonatal gerbils; however, these parameters approximate adult values by 8 weeks of age. The presence of stippled red cells and reticulocytes at levels higher than those of most other domestic rodent species may be caused by the short lifespan of erythrocytes in gerbils (approximately 9–10 days), which necessitates a continuous hyperactive state of erythropoiesis.

Hematologic features in other rodents

Features of hematology among the other rodents, such as chinchillas, resemble those of rats and mice. The blood volume of the Syrian hamster is between 65 and 80 mL per kilogram of body weight, of which 1 mL

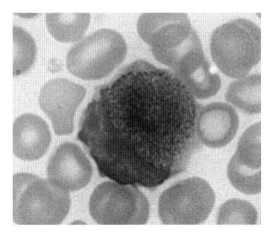

Fig. 6. Foa-Kurloff cell with Kurloff's body inclusion. This type of cell is unique to the guinea pig.

can be drawn safely during a single collection. White blood cell (WBC) counts decline during hibernation and a pronounced leukocytosis (neutrophilia) can be observed in hamsters waking from hibernative periods. Polychromasia is a normal finding in blood films of healthy animals and Howell-Jolly bodies are common. Neutrophils in chinchillas are usually hypersegmented.

White blood cell estimation

A small drop of blood is required to make an appropriate blood smear film for evaluation, either being sent to a diagnostic laboratory for the CBC or for in-house WBC estimation and cell differential counts. Skill is required to make thin smears with a nicely feathered edge or results can be erroneous. When estimating, the numbers of leukocytes per ×40 objective from at least five fields are counted on a stained blood smear. The average number of leukocytes is then multiplied by 1000 to make an estimated total white cell count. When performed, this number should be compared with the actual cell count, depending on the method used to obtain the overall WBC.

Bone marrow evaluation

Indications for bone marrow analysis, cytologic evaluation, methods of collection and smear preparation, and unique morphologic features of bone marrow cells are discussed. The following information relates primarily to bone marrow collection in the rat, but procedures are applicable to most rodent species.

In clinical practice, bone marrow examination is recommended when a primary or secondary hematologic disorder is present that cannot be explained by peripheral blood examination alone. These conditions include nonregenerative anemia, thrombocytopenias, gammopathy, lymphoproliferative disorders (eg, leukemia), or suspect neoplasia. Bone marrow evaluation also is indicated for staging certain malignancies (lymphoma, mast cell tumors) or investigating abnormalities such as unexplained fever or hypercalcemia.

Evaluation of the hematopoietic system also should include histologic examination of bone marrow and assessment of other hematopoietic organs (ie, spleen, lymph nodes). It is important to be familiar with the normal cytology of rat bone marrow so that alterations can be recognized and accurately interpreted. Bone marrow evaluation is frequently used in biomedical research to determine hematotoxicity of experimental drugs and other toxicologic analysis.

The most common site for sampling in small exotic mammals is the proximal femur, although the proximal tibia, proximal humerus, and the ileum can be used depending on the patient size.

General anesthesia is required to facilitate restraint and minimize risk to the patient. Infiltration of the sampling site with a local anesthetic such as

2% lidocaine is also important. The patient is placed in lateral recumbency and the hair overlying the greater trochanter shaved. The site is then surgically prepared and a small stab incision is made through the skin with a scalpel blade. A spinal needle with stylet in place is advanced and seated into the medullary cavity by rotating in a clockwise-counterclockwise manner.

Once properly seated, the stylet can be removed and a syringe attached to the hub. Negative pressure is applied until blood appears and marrow is aspirated into the hub. Excessive negative pressure should be avoided, because peripheral blood artifact may make interpretation difficult. After collection the sample is placed into EDTA and slides are prepared before clotting. A few drops of a 10% EDTA solution can be placed in the syringe before aspiration to prevent clotting.

Bone marrow films are best made by placing a drop of marrow on a glass slide, placing another slide on top with little to no pressure, and then pulling the slides apart after the drop has spread. Slides are then allowed to air dry before staining. In clinical practice, stains such as Wright's-Giemsa and rapid hematologic stains commonly are used. Bone marrow smears require more staining time than blood smears, because marrow smears are thicker and the material is unevenly distributed. Special stains can be performed on unstained slides. Because rat bone marrow contains a large number of mast cells, free mast cell granules from disrupted cells also may be seen in the background.

Examination of bone marrow should include determination of the myeloid:erythroid (M:E) ratio. The normal M:E ratio varies with species but is generally between 0.5:1 and 3:1. The normal ratio for the rat ranges from 1.16:1 to 1.36:1, for mice and gerbils it is 0.75:1 to 2.35:1, and for guinea pigs it is between 1.5:1 and 1.9:1 [5,6].

The maturation index (proliferation index; the ratio of proliferating to nonproliferating cells) has been calculated for rats and seems to be stable. This value is useful for characterizing abnormalities of maturation and verifying subjective interpretations of ineffective hematopoiesis. The accuracy of these calculations can be ensured only when the bone marrow examinations are performed on high-quality smears.

Response in disease

Hypoplasia of the bone marrow can result from chemical toxicity, infectious disease, estrogen toxicity, myelofibrosis, or immune-mediated disorders. The lack of cells from all of the cell lines is an indication of bone marrow aplasia. Most cases in domestic animals relate to immunosuppressive therapy or immune-mediated disease.

Hyperplasia of the marrow can occur as a regenerative response to the peripheral loss of cells. The response may be either myeloid or erythroid, depending on the type of cell loss. Hyperplasia can also result from neoplastic disorders, such as lymphoproliferative or myeloproliferative diseases.

Disorders of hematology

Anemia is represented by a low red blood cell count or hematocrit that falls below the reference range for a given species. An uncommon cause of hemolytic anemia could be blood parasites, although these are rarely seen in pet rodents. Chronic blood loss could also relate to heavy lice infestations sometimes observed in rats and guinea pigs.

Cavian leukemia/type C retrovirus

Lymphosarcoma is the most common type of neoplasia affecting guinea pigs and can be caused by a retrovirus. Diagnosis is based on results of the CBC count and cytologic examination of aspirates from lymph nodes of guinea pigs with peripheral lymphadenopathy. Leukemic guinea pigs often show a severe leukocytosis with counts of 25 to 500 $\times$ 10^3 cells/mm^3 [7] (the author has seen lymphocyte counts more than $90 \times 10^3/\mu$L, with differential counts of greater than 90% lymphocytes and lymphoblasts present in peripheral circulation). Prognosis is grave and most succumb within 4 weeks. Some guinea pigs have experienced response to chemotherapy; however, this therapy is not commonly performed because of client choice, difficulty, and patient sensitivity to administration of chemotherapy agents [8].

Guinea pigs experimentally infected with *Trixacarus caviae* (guinea pig mange mite) developed a heterophilia, monocytosis, eosinophilia, and basophilia [9]. Guinea pigs have also developed eosinophilia in response to *Treponema pallidum* (syphilis) infections (Appendix 1) [10].

Summary

Veterinarians who treat rodents will find clinical practice more rewarding when performing appropriate diagnostic evaluation that includes blood tests. Preanesthetic screening, as performed in all other companion animals, will also lead to better pre- and postoperative care and minimize mortality. Providing clients with better prognostic information will help ameliorate unexplainable deaths and improve the chances of helping more pets. It will also help advance veterinary medicine while enhancing veterinarians' vital relationships with caring pet owners.

Appendix 1

Recommended reading

Campbell TW. Mammalian hematology: laboratory animals and miscellaneous species. In: Thrall MA, editor. Veterinary hematology and clinical chemistry. 1st edition. Lippincott Williams and Wilkins, 2004. p. 211–224.

Campbell TW, Ellis CK. Avian and exotic animal hematology and cytology. 3rd edition. Ames (IA): Blackwell Publishing; 2007.

Moore DM. Hematology of rabbits and hematology of the guinea pig. In: Feldman BF, Zinkl JG, Jain NC, editors. Schlam's veterinary hematology. 5th edition. Lippincott Williams & Wilkins; 2000. p. 1100–1110.

Quesenberry KE, Carpenter JW, editors. Ferrets, rabbits, and rodents: clinical medicine and surgery. 2nd edition. St Louis (MO): Saunders.

References

[1] Wiedmeyer CE, Ruben D, Franklin C. Complete blood count, clinical chemistry, and serology profile by using a single tube of whole blood from mice. J Am Assoc Lab Anim Sci 2007;46(2):59–64.

[2] Reuter RE. Venipuncture in the guinea pig. Lab Anim Sci 1987;37:245–6.

[3] Hem A, Smith AJ, Solberg P. Saphenous vein puncture for blood sampling of the mouse, rat, hamster, gerbil, guinea pig, ferret and mink. Lab Anim 1998;32:364–8.

[4] Sisk DB. Physiology. In: Wagner JE, Manning PJ, editors. The biology of the guinea pig. New York: Academic Press; 1976. p. 63–92.

[5] Harris RS, Herdan G, Ancill RJ, et al. A quantitative comparison of the nucleated cells in the right and left humeral bone marrow of the guinea pig. Blood 1954;9:374–8.

[6] Dineen JK, Adams DB. The effect of long term lymphatic drainage on the lympho-myeloid system in the guinea pig. Immunology 1970;19:11–30.

[7] Collins B. Common diseases and medical management of rodents and lagomorphs. In: Jacobson ER, Kolias GV, editors. Exotic animals. New York: Churchill Livingstone; 1988. p. 261–316.

[8] Manning PJ, Wagner JE, Harkness JE. Biology and diseases of guinea pigs. In: Fox JG, Cohen BJ, Loew FM, editors. Laboratory animal medicine. Orlando (FL): Academic Press; 1984. p. 149–81.

[9] Rothwell TLW, Pope SE, Rajczyk ZK, et al. Haematological and pathological responses to experimental *Trixacarus caviae* infection in guinea pigs. J Comp Pathol 1991;104:179–85.

[10] Wicher V, Scarozza AM, Ramsingh AI, et al. Cytokine gene expression in skin of susceptible guinea-pig infected with *Treponema pallidum*. Immunology 1998;95:242–7.

VETERINARY
CLINICS
Exotic Animal Practice

ELSEVIER
SAUNDERS

Vet Clin Exot Anim 11 (2008) 535–550

Ferret Hematology
and Related Disorders

Linda J. Siperstein, DVM

VCA Wakefield Animal Hospital, 19 Main Street, Wakefield, MA 01880, USA

Although the staying power of the pet ferret (*Mustela putorius furo*) in the United States may have been in question 10 years ago, by all current indications, this animal's popularity is not in any danger. Fortunately, our understanding of these exotic animals as pets and as patients has grown over the years. Research and publication on the subject of ferret hematology, however, has been somewhat limited in the past 10 years. This article summarizes previous publications on this subject, mentions some clinical techniques used by the author's own hospital, outlines several common diseases and their effect on the hemogram, and discusses the need for further research.

Restraint

When working with exotic species, understanding proper restraint is often half the battle. For physical examinations, "scruffing" a ferret and allowing the patient to simply hang loosely causes most ferrets to relax (and yawn) for the entirety of the examination. The same principles can be used when taking blood samples; only the position of the patient changes.

Although anesthesia guarantees a more cooperative patient, it is not necessary in most cases. Also, anesthesia affects hematologic values, making interpretation of blood from anesthetized patients difficult. These effects are described later in this article.

Several restraint techniques have been described for phlebotomy in which larger volumes (1–3 mL) are needed. One technique involves scruffing the ferret in a hanging position, wrapping it in a towel, and then placing the toweled ferret in dorsal recumbency for cranial vena cava (CVC) or jugular venipuncture (Fig. 1). Alternatively, for jugular venipuncture, the ferret is

E-mail address: dr.siperstein@yahoo.com

1094-9194/08/$ - see front matter © 2008 Elsevier Inc. All rights reserved.
doi:10.1016/j.cvex.2008.03.009   *vetexotic.theclinics.com*

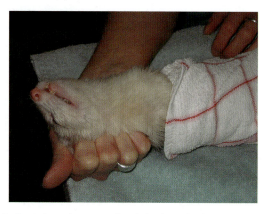

Fig. 1. Restraint using a towel and the ferret in dorsal recumbency.

held over the edge of a table with the neck dorsoflexed, as in a cat (Fig. 2). The technique that the author uses at her practice involves simply placing the ferret in dorsal recumbency and scruffing the patient such that the head and neck are as flat as possible to the table. The front legs are gently extended caudally (Fig. 3). If needed, a second technician restrains the

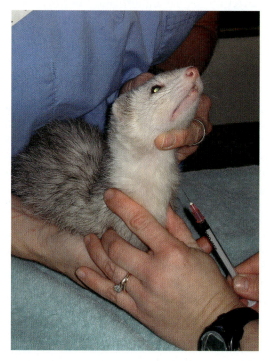

Fig. 2. Restraint as in the cat, with the ferret's head dorsoflexed.

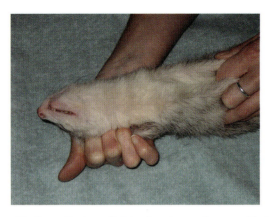

Fig. 3. Restraint with the patient scruffed in dorsal recumbency, with the legs extended caudally.

caudal aspect of the patient to prevent wiggling. Because the author draws almost all blood samples from the CVC and this position provides excellent access to the neck, this technique has proved ideal for the author's purposes.

Phlebotomy

The total blood volume in the ferret is approximately 6% of the body weight. It is generally safe, therefore, to draw as much as 6 mL from a 1-kg ferret [1]. Care should be taken in the anemic patient only to draw as much blood as is needed, however. In the case of most laboratory panels, a 1-mL sample is sufficient to yield accurate results. Microtainer (Becton Dickinson and Company, Franklin Lakes, New Jersey) collection tubes are available from most laboratories that perform blood work on exotics.

For collection of small blood volumes, the lateral saphenous or cephalic vein is adequate (Fig. 4). If it is necessary to visualize the vein, the area can be shaved. Alternatively, applying alcohol to wet the fur may provide suffi-cient exposure. Use of the caudal tail artery or vein has been described but is more painful and, given other options, not necessary.

For larger volumes of blood (1–3 mL), the CVC or the jugular vein is pre-ferred [2]. Restraint techniques, as described previously, allow good access to these sites. In the past, the CVC was discouraged as a venipuncture site because of "inherently greater risks" without an explanation of those risks [3]. As Capello [1] describes, however, this technique is actually useful and safe, not only for the ferret but for many other small mammals. Given the more caudal location of the heart in the ferret, the clinician should not be concerned about accidental cardiac puncture. At the author's prac-tice, she draws from the CVC almost exclusively for blood samples in ferret patients, with consistent success and no complications. To access the CVC,

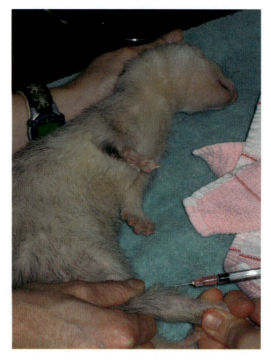

Fig. 4. Venipuncture from the lateral saphenous vein.

the animal is held in dorsal recumbency and scruffed (as described previously) with an assistant holding the animal still. The patients seem to settle
into this position quickly. If alcohol is applied, most ferrets startle momen-
tarily; therefore, the author applies alcohol before she is ready for the blood
draw. Once the patient has settled down, she then places it in position for
phlebotomy. A 1-inch 25- or 27-gauge needle is placed at the thoracic notch
(Figs. 5 and 6) and inserted at an angle of 45° to the body, directed toward
the rear leg opposite from the hub. The needle is then slowly withdrawn until blood is seen in the hub. Although this blind technique requires a little
practice (it can be helpful for the beginner to practice on compliant ferrets
or on those already anesthetized for other purposes), once mastered, it is
quick, dependable, and safe.

As previously described, jugular venipuncture is also an option with the
ferret in dorsal recumbency, or in ventral recumbency with the head extended as in the cat. Shaving of the neck can aid in better visualization of
the jugular vein. (Bear in mind that ferrets suspected of adrenal tumors
may be slow to regrow fur in shaved areas.) The one disadvantage of using
the jugular vein for venipuncture is the flat thin nature of the vessel, which
can make it difficult to maintain the needle within the vessel lumen [1].

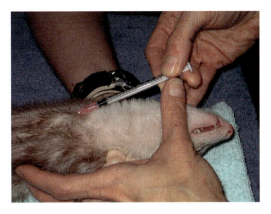

Fig. 5. Positioned for venipuncture from the CVC.

Red blood cell and white blood cell morphology

The hematocrit and red blood cell (RBC) values for adult ferrets are generally higher than the values found in dogs and cats. In addition, the lifespan of the RBC is shorter in the ferret than in the dog or cat, resulting in increased polychromasia (Patty Ewing, DVM, MS, DACVP, Department of Pathology, Angell Animal Medical Center, Boston, MA, personal communication, 2008).

On the differential count, neutrophils are the predominant leukocyte and contain polychromatic granules. Eosinophils have a single or bilobed

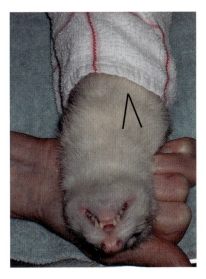

Fig. 6. Landmarks for thoracic notch, venipuncture from CVC.

nucleus, basophils are described as segmented, and monocytes are usually vacuolated in appearance [4].

By way of comparison with the dog and cat, ferret neutrophils have small pale-red granules that are not usually visible or are less prominent than those of cat or dog neutrophils. Ferret eosinophil granules are rounder, unlike the rod-shaped granules of the cat eosinophil. In addition, ferret eosinophil granules are smaller and brighter red than in the dog. Ferret basophils are similar in appearance to dog basophils, whereas cat basophils, by comparison, have a paler lavender appearance to the granules (Patty Ewing, DVM, MS, DACVP, Department of Pathology, Angell Animal Medical Center, Boston, MA, personal communication, 2008) (Figs. 7–10).

Interpretation of the hemogram

Although hematologic values in the ferret are often referred to as similar to those in other mammals, specifically other domestic carnivores, it is important to recognize several important differences. In general, the hematocrit, hemoglobin, and total erythrocyte and reticulocyte counts are higher than in the dog or cat [5]. White blood cell (WBC) counts tend to be low in ferrets; therefore, the clinician must be careful not to misinterpret counts in the range from 3000 to 4000 WBCs/μL as leukopenias. In addition, WBC responses seem to be rare in disease situations; left shifts are uncommon in the ferret [6]. Differences in normal ranges are seen between albino and fitch ferrets and between male and female ferrets (Table 1).

Kawasaki [6] reports the mean normal differential lymphocyte count in ferrets as 35%, with an absolute count of 3500 WBCs/μL as the upper limit of the normal range. He proposes that in cases of chronic lymphocytosis (greater than 3500 WBCs/μL), one should consider the following interpretations: that this count is normal for the patient, that the patient is demonstrating chronic antigenic stimulation as with viral infection, or that this

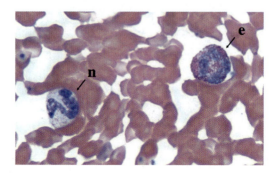

Fig. 7. Ferret eosinophil (e) and neutrophil (n). (*Courtesy of* Dr. Patty Ewing, Boston, MA.)

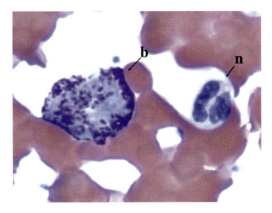

Fig. 8. Ferret basophil (b) and neutrophil (n). (*Courtesy of* Dr. Patty Ewing, Boston, MA.)

represents evidence of "early lymphosarcoma or lymphoproliferative disorder." When reading blood smears, heavier lymphocytes can sometimes be pushed to one area, and therefore may falsely elevate the lymphocyte count [6].

As in most mammals, elevations in eosinophils can suggest allergic disease (lung disease or skin allergies) or parasitic disease, such as ferret heartworm infection. A peripheral eosinophilia can also result from eosinophilic gastroenteritis, a condition not uncommon in the ferret [6].

If anemia is present, the clinician should consider any cause of anemia seen in other mammals. The ferret is particularly prone to certain conditions; therefore, one should give particular consideration to rule-outs, such as lymphoma, adrenal tumors, hyperestrogenism, gastric ulcers, infection, or hepatic or renal disease [6].

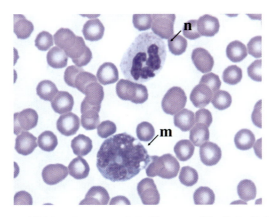

Fig. 9. Ferret neutrophil (n) and monocyte (m). (*Courtesy of* Dr. Patty Ewing, Boston, MA.)

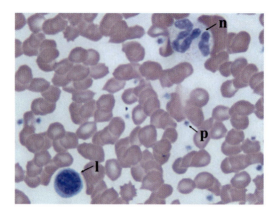

Fig. 10. Ferret neutrophil (n), platelets (p), and small lymphocyte (l). (*Courtesy of* Dr. Patty Ewing, Boston, MA.)

Factors affecting the normal hemogram

Age

Young ferrets demonstrate differences in their hemogram compared with their adult counterparts, with some additional distinctions between male and female ferrets. In a study at Oklahoma State University, blood samples were drawn over time to determine age-related changes in young ferrets from 12 to 18 weeks in female ferrets and from 12 to 47 weeks in male ferrets

Table 1
Hematologic values of ferrets

Measurements	Albino ferrets		Fitch ferrets	
	Male	Female	Male	Female
PCV (%)	55 (44–61)	49 (42–55)	43 (36–50)	48 (47–51)
RBCs (10^6 cells/μL)	10.2 (7.3–12.2)	8.1 (6.8–9.8)	—	—
Hemoglobin (g/dL)	17.8 (16.3–18.2)	16.2 (14.8–17.4)	14.3 (12.0–16.3)	15.9 (15.2–17.4)
WBCs (10^3 cells/μL)	9.7 (4.4–19.1)	10.5 (4.0–18.2)	11.3 (7.7–15.4)	5.9 (2.5–8.6)
Neutrophils (%)	57 (11–82)	60 (43–84)	40 (24–78)	31 (12–41)
Band cells (%)	—	—	0.9 (0–2.2)	1.7 (0–4.2)
Lymphocytes (%)	36 (12–54)[a]	33 (12–50)	50 (28–69)	58 (25–95)
Monocytes (%)	4 (0–9)	4 (2–8)	6.6 (3.4–8.2)	4.5 (1.7–6.3)
Eosinophils (%)	2 (0–7)	3 (0–5)	2 (0–7)	4 (1–9)
Basophils (%)	0.1 (0–2)	0.2 (0–1)	0.7 (0–2.7)	0.8 (0–2.9)
Platelets (10^3 cells/μL)	453 (297–730)	545 (310–910)	—	—
Reticulocytes (%)	4 (1–12)	5 (2–14)	—	—

[a] May be as high as 75% in young ferrets.

Data from Carpenter J. Exotic animal formulary. 3rd edition. St. Louis (MO): Elsevier Saunders; 2005. p. 466.

(female ferrets were taken out of the study by approximately 18 weeks because of pregnancy). In male ferrets, the study showed an age-related increase in RBC counts, hemoglobin, packed cell volume (PCV), and segmented neutrophils, and a decrease in lymphocytes from 12 to 47 weeks. In female ferrets, an age-related increase in segmented neutrophils and a decrease in PCV and lymphocytes were documented from 12 to 18 weeks of age [7]. Generally speaking, ferrets younger than 5 to 7 months of age normally can have lymphocytes as the predominant cell type on their differential count and age- and gender-dependent changes in the PCV [6]. Therefore, one must avoid misinterpretation of the hemogram of young ferrets.

Isofluorane

Whereas blood samples can be drawn in the anesthetized ferret, these results can be difficult to interpret. WBC counts are only somewhat decreased by isofluorane; however, the hematocrit, RBC count, and hemoglobin concentrations are abruptly and significantly decreased. According to Marini and colleagues [8], the hematocrit seems to be decreased by approximately 36%. The physiologic mechanisms of these alterations were studied by Marini and colleagues [8], using technetium 99m-labeled RBCs to determine that isoflurane causes splenic sequestration of RBCs. They also demonstrated partial reversal of this effect by injecting phenylephrine. The conclusion of the study points out that blood samples taken in anesthetized ferrets must be interpreted with caution. If the safety of the patient would be compromised by attempting phlebotomy in an awake ferret, anesthesia should be considered.

Disorders of the ferret and their effect on the hemogram

Several disease conditions can result in alterations of the ferret hemogram. Although some of these conditions are the same as those included in the rule-out list of any dog or cat, certain conditions are particularly prevalent in ferrets. Without delving into a complete discussion of ferret diseases, the topics addressed here are specifically relevant to changes in the ferret RBC and WBC counts.

Estrous

Female ferrets are seasonally polyestrous-induced ovulators and are at risk of hyperestrogenism if ovulation does not occur. Signs of normal estrous may include an enlarged vulva and vulvar discharge. Most ferrets in the United States are spayed or neutered before entering the pet trade. In the case of the unspayed ferret or spayed ferrets with ovarian remnants, however, hyperestrogenism with resulting bone marrow hypoplasia is fatal unless the ferret ovulates. In one study of the effects of estrus in ferrets, hematologic findings included thrombocytopenia, granulocytopenia, and hypocellularity of the bone marrow. Aplastic anemia was present in 50% of the animals, with reduction in hematopoiesis in the spleen. Hemorrhagic anemia attributable to thrombocytopenia was the most common cause of death, with the ferrets most commonly bleeding into the skin, buccal mucosa, and gastrointestinal (GI) tract. In this study, deaths began within 2 months of onset of estrus [9].

Treatment of female ferrets that have hyperestrogenism depends on the severity of the disease and includes supportive care (subcutaneous or intravenous fluids, syringe feeding, and antibiotics, if indicated) and blood transfusion if the PCV drops to less than 15% to 20%. The patient should be spayed once stable enough for surgery.

Adrenal disease

Clinically, ferrets that have adrenal disease may present with a progressive alopecia, pruritus, and an enlarged vulva in the female ferret or dysuria, stranguria, or urinary blockage in some male ferrets. The results of a complete blood cell count (CBC) are usually normal; however, a nonregenerative anemia can occur. This anemia is rarely as severe as in unspayed female ferrets that have prolonged estrus and its resulting hyperestrogenism. Nevertheless, if the patient is a spayed female ferret demonstrating a nonregenerative anemia, the differential diagnosis should include an ovarian remnant.

Diagnosis of adrenal disease can be confirmed with ultrasound of the adrenal glands. Treatment options include surgical removal of the diseased adrenal gland or initiation of leuprolide acetate (Lupron) injections.

Although removal of the left adrenal gland is fairly straightforward, the right adrenal gland is located immediately adjacent to the caudal vena cava and removal of this gland requires an experienced surgeon.

At the author's practice, ferrets receiving leuprolide acetate injections are given 100 μg intramuscularly every 4 weeks. Initially, most ferrets do not show clinical improvement until after the second injection. The author purchases human leuprolide acetate, makes up 100-μg/0.2-mL syringes, and keeps these frozen until use. (Care must be taken while handling this drug; wear gloves.) If a ferret's response to monthly treatments becomes unsatisfactory, the author gives injections every 3 weeks.

Any treatment choices are preceded by, or given concurrently with, appropriate supportive care. Treatment options are also dictated by the owner's financial abilities, whether only one or both adrenal glands are affected, and the overall health status of the ferret. Once the disease is controlled, a previously abnormal hemogram should return to normal [10,11].

Insulinoma

Pancreatic islet cell tumors are common in ferrets around the age of 4 to 5 years and result from lack of a proper feedback mechanism on the part of the tumor cells, which, in turn, results in hypoglycemia. Symptoms may include lethargy, weakness, ataxia, and eventually collapse or seizures. Weight loss and vomiting may also be noted, and some animals paw at the mouth. In many cases, patients may only show intermittent brief episodes of weakness. At the author's practice, a ferret demonstrating any of these clinical signs and a blood glucose level less than 60 to 65 mg/dL is presumed to have insulinoma unless another cause is determined.

On the CBC, leukocytosis, neutrophilia, and monocytosis are sometimes present, but the hemogram may be entirely normal until the patient becomes severely ill.

Surgical removal of individual tumors or a partial pancreatectomy is usually the treatment of choice; however, medical management with prednisone alone or in conjunction with diazoxide (Proglycem) is an option for older ferrets or when owners cannot afford surgery. Both of these medications can be acquired from a compounding pharmacy, allowing for more practical dosing. Patients at the author's practice are usually started on prednisone at a dosage of 0.5 mg/kg divided twice daily, and slowly increased (as high as 4 mg/kg divided twice daily) until clinical signs resolve and the blood glucose is normal or, in the author's experience, as close to normal as can be achieved. Blood glucose in a stable patient may be checked every 1 to 2 weeks to assess response to treatment. The author adds diazoxide if prednisone alone is not sufficient, starting at a dose of 5 to 10 mg/kg, and increasing slowly up to 30 mg/kg. When adding diazoxide, the author decreases prednisone to half of the current dose.

Surgery is not curative but rather slows or stops the progression of the disease. This lack of a true cure is partially attributable to the fact that insulinoma of the ferret most commonly presents in the form of microtumors spread throughout the pancreas. Medical management, when effective, controls the clinical signs of the hypoglycemia; however, unlike surgery, it does not stop progression of the tumor. Once better controlled, however, any abnormalities in the hemogram should resolve temporarily [10–12].

Lymphoma

Along with adrenal disease and pancreatic islet cell tumors, lymphoma is one of the most common diseases seen in ferrets. Clinical signs are generally nonspecific, and may include lethargy, anorexia, and weight loss. Depending on organs affected, clients may also note vomiting, diarrhea, labored breathing, pruritus or dermatitis, or paresis. Signs can sometimes wax and wane, although some ferrets may be asymptomatic for years. Physical examination may reveal enlarged peripheral lymph nodes, weight loss, a noncompressible cranial thorax, dyspnea, splenic enlargement, or an abdominal mass. For those unaccustomed to seeing pet ferrets, it is important to bear in mind that the lymph nodes of normal ferrets can be surrounded by fat, which should not be mistaken for lymph node enlargement.

On the CBC, ferrets with lymphoma commonly exhibit anemia, a relative or absolute lymphocytosis, and occasionally, neutropenia and thrombocytopenia [6]. In young ferrets, lymphocytosis is more common, whereas lymphopenias are seen more often in older ferrets [13]. It is important to note, however, that not all ferrets with lymphoma demonstrate abnormalities of their lymphocyte count.

As in cats and dogs, radiographs, ultrasound, bone marrow aspirate, and lymph node biopsy can aid in diagnosis of lymphoma. Temporary remission is sometimes achieved using one of the various combination chemotherapy protocols described in the literature. If owners do not elect combination chemotherapy, prednisone alone can achieve remission; however, such remission is usually of shorter duration. Use of prednisone for preexisting diseases, such as insulinoma, may diminish the patient's response to subsequent chemotherapy protocols. The CBC is important in assessing response to treatment and any adverse reaction to chemotherapy drugs [13–15].

Eosinophilic gastroenteritis

Eosinophilic gastroenteritis is a GI disease involving infiltration of the GI muscosa by eosinophils. This infiltration causes inflammation of the mucosa and can lead to diarrhea with or without mucus or blood, anorexia, vomiting, and weight loss. Although allergy and parasitism have been proposed as causes of eosinophilic gastroenteritis, the underlying cause remains unknown [16,17]. Diagnosis is usually made on the basis of gastric or intestinal biopsy.

The hemogram of ferrets with eosinophilic gastroenteritis may reveal an eosinophilia as high as 35%, [18]; however, not all ferrets demonstrate eosinophilia. Eosinophilic gastroenteritis should be on the rule-out list for any ferret with an elevated eosinophil count or chronic diarrhea with or without eosinophilia on the CBC. Other rule-outs should include dietary indiscretion, gastric ulcers, GI foreign body, any cause of inflammatory bowel disease (IBD), viral or bacterial infection, parasitism, or lymphosarcoma [18].

Treatment of eosinophilic gastroenteritis should begin by addressing any dehydration and vomiting. Depending on the severity of dehydration from vomiting or diarrhea, subcutaneous or intravenous fluids are administered. Antibiotics, such as metronidazole (Flagyl) may be helpful in controlling diarrhea, and sucralfate (Carafate) can be added for any GI bleeding. If vomiting has resolved, syringe feeding with Carnivore Care (Oxbow Hay Company, Murdock, Nebraska) can help to stimulate appetite. The disease is usually controlled with prednisone, and dosing may be tapered until a therapeutic dose is found. Concurrent use of antibiotics may be indicated to prevent secondary bacterial infection. Unfortunately, some ferrets do not respond to prednisone, or signs recur once the dose is decreased. The prognosis is good for ferrets that respond well to prednisone [18].

Addressing disease conditions

Although some specific diseases are discussed in this article, any condition resulting in severe illness can lead to a lowered PCV, risk of infection, or insult to the coagulation pathway. As with any other patient, when indicated, blood transfusion, antibiotics, fluid support, and treatment of the specific disease should be administered.

Blood groups

Most mammals demonstrate blood groups that lead to an antibody response when the patient is not cross-matched for transfusion or if transfused more than once. In the case of the ferret, there seem to be no blood groups or the ferret's antigen system is too weak to respond to blood transfusion. As a result, transfusion in the ferret does not require cross-matching, and any available and appropriate (healthy) blood donor is an acceptable source. In addition, if repeated transfusions are necessary, the clinician is not faced with the same risks (eg, antigenic response, rejection, death) seen in other mammalian patients [19]. In one documented case, a female ferret that had estrus-induced anemia was given 13 transfusions from three unrelated donors over approximately 5 months with no apparent transfusion reaction [20].

Blood transfusions

When the PCV decreases to less than 25% and clinical signs warrant, a blood transfusion may be indicated [2]. For the purposes of blood transfusion, blood can be drawn from the CVC or the jugular vein using a butterfly catheter. A male adult ferret (with a normal PCV) is ideal, because male ferrets are generally larger and more blood can safely be drawn.

With the donor anesthetized, blood is collected into a syringe with 1 mL of the anticoagulant acid citrate dextrose per 6 mL of blood [2]. The blood can then be administered immediately to the recipient patient though a 21- or 22-gauge catheter into the jugular vein or using an intraosseous catheter over a period of 5 to 10 minutes [3,21]. As already discussed, 6 to 10 mL of blood can be safely drawn from the donor, depending on the donor's weight. As with blood transfusion in any animal, good sterile technique should be used and a single clean stick is important to prevent clotting of the sample. Replacement of blood with warm intravenous fluids can prevent hypotension in the donor [21].

Coagulation times

Assessment of coagulation is performed much as in the cat or dog, with consideration of the ferret's size and limitations on how much blood can safely be removed from this small patient.

Prothrombin time (PT) and activated partial thromboplastin time (APTT) can be useful in the assessment of extrinsic and intrinsic coagulation pathways. Blood is collected in a sodium citrate tube and submitted to the laboratory. Because a patient with a bleeding disorder may be compromised by a large blood draw for these tests, using smaller samples is important. Small "exotics" sodium citrate tubes, such as a Microtainer, should be available from any laboratory that performs blood work on exotic species. Carpenter's *Exotic Animal Formulary* [22] lists a normal PT of 8.0 to 16.5 seconds and a normal APTT of 16 to 25 seconds.

Coagulation can be affected by low platelets, the effects of which may not be immediately apparent on the PT or APTT. The clinician can assess clotting using a buccal mucosal bleeding time (BMBT); however, this test is more easily performed in the anesthetized ferret [21].

Bone marrow collection

Bone marrow collection can aid in assessment of anemias, thrombocytopenias, pancytopenias, proliferative abnormalities, and hematopoietic malignancies. The best sites for collection in the ferret are the proximal femur, the iliac crest, and the humerus. For the femur, the patient is anesthetized and aseptically prepared, and a skin incision is made over the greater trochanter. As in other species, the femur is stabilized while inserting a spinal needle (1.5-inch, 20-gauge) into the shaft of the bone, starting just medial to the greater trochanter. By rotating the needle and applying gentle pressure, the needle is advanced into the marrow cavity. The stylet is removed, a 6-mL syringe is attached, and a marrow sample is aspirated into the syringe. Once the sample is visualized in the syringe, stop aspiration right away and prepare slides quickly. Preparation of slides is performed as in the dog or cat, using two slides to spread the spicules across the slide. Provide the pathologist with at least four slides for examination [2].

Need for further research

Although we have made great strides in understanding our ferret patients and their anatomy and physiology, a great deal is still not well understood that could help us to treat the ailing patient better. We continue to struggle with understanding the mechanisms responsible for adrenal disease; therefore, we still do not know how to prevent this common (in the United States) problem in our patients. Any clinician who sees ferrets would love to know how to make adrenal disease and pancreatic islet cell tumors diseases of the past. At one time, we did not know that adding taurine to a cat's diet could all but eliminate dilated cardiomyopathy from our lineup of feline diseases. Perhaps some of our more frustrating ferret conditions may be similarly demystified in the not-too-distant future.

Summary

The ferret has proved itself to be a companionable and friendly patient, pet, and family member, and we should expect that its popularity is not likely to wane any time soon. The more that research is funded and clinicians are willing to share their observations and case findings, the more we can add to our knowledge of this sometimes challenging patient.

Acknowledgments

The author thanks Kristin Haroutunian for allowing Georgie and Joey to pose for the photographs, the technicians at the VCA Wakefield Animal Hospital for their assistance in taking these photographs, Dr. Patty Ewing for her extraordinary clinical pathology support, and Dr. Gary R. Cook and Dr. Laurie Siperstein-Cook for their insight.

References

[1] Capello V. Application of the cranial vena cava venipuncture technique to small exotic mammals. Seminars in avian and exotic pet medicine 1997;6(1):51–5.

[2] Quesenberry K, Orcutt C. Basic approach to veterinary care. In: Quesenberry K, Carpenter J, editors. Ferrets, rabbits, and rodents. 2nd edition. Missouri (MO): Saunders; 2003. p. 13–24.

[3] Brown S. Clinical techniques in domestic ferrets. Seminars in avian and exotic pet medicine 1997;6(2):75–85.

[4] Moore D. Hematology of the ferret. In: Feldman B, Zinkl J, Jain N, editors. Schalm's veterinary hematology. 5th edition. Philadelphia: Lippincott Williams and Wilkins; 2000. p. 1096–9.

[5] Marini R, Otto G, Erdman S, et al. Biology and diseases of ferrets. In: Fox J, Anderson L, Loew F, et al, editors. Laboratory animal medicine. London: Academic Press; 2002. p. 483–517.

[6] Kawasaki T. Normal parameters and laboratory interpretation of disease states in the domestic ferret. Seminars in avian and exotic pet medicine 1994;3(1):40–7.

[7] Hoover J, Baldwin C. Changes in physiologic and clinicopathologic values in domestic ferrets from 12–47 weeks of age. Companion animal practice 1988;2(1):40–4.

[8] Marini R, Callahan R, Jackson L, et al. Distribution of technetium 99m-labeled red blood cells during isoflurane anesthesia in ferrets. Am J Vet Res 1997;58(7):781–5.

[9] Sherill A, Gorham J. Bone marrow hypoplasia associated with estrus in ferrets. J Am Assoc Lab Anim Sci 1985;35(1):280–6.

[10] Fox J, Marini R. Diseases of the endocrine system. In: Fox J, editor. Biology and diseases of the ferret. 2nd edition. Baltimore (MD): Williams & Wilkins; 1998. p. 291–305.

[11] Quesenberry K, Rosenthal K. Endocrine diseases. In: Quesenberry K, Carpenter J, editors. Ferrets, rabbits, and rodents. 2nd edition. Missouri (MO): Saunders; 2003. p. 79–90.

[12] Oglesbee B. Insulinoma. In: Oglesbee B, editor. The 5-minute veterinary consult ferret and rabbit. Iowa (IA): Blackwell Publishing; 2006. p. 85–7.

[13] Erdman S, Xiantang L, Fox J. Hematopoietic diseases. In: Fox J, editor. Biology and diseases of the ferret. 2nd edition. Baltimore (MD): Williams & Wilkins; 1998. p. 231–46.

[14] Williams B, Weiss C. Neoplasia. In: Quesenberry K, Carpenter J, editors. Ferrets, rabbits, and rodents. 2nd edition. Missouri (MO): Saunders; 2003. p. 91–106.

[15] Oglesbee B. Lymphosarcoma. In: Oglesbee B, editor. The 5-minute veterinary consult ferret and rabbit. Iowa (IA): Blackwell Publishing; 2006. p. 94–6.

[16] Fazakas S. Eosinophilic gastroenteritis in a domestic ferret. Can Vet J 2000;41:707–9.

[17] Palley L, Fox J. Eosinophilic gastroenteritis in the ferret. In: Kirk's current veterinary therapy XI: small animal practice. Philadelphia: WB Saunders; 1992. p. 1182–4.

[18] Fox J. Diseases of the gastrointestinal system. In: Fox J, editor. Biology and diseases of the ferret. 2nd edition. Baltimore (MD): Williams & Wilkins; 1998. p. 273–90.

[19] Manning D, Bell J. Lack of detectable blood groups in domestic ferrets: implications for transfusion. J Am Vet Med Assoc 1990;197(1):84–6.

[20] Ryland LM. Remission of estrus-associated anemia following ovariohysterectomy and multiple blood transfusions in a ferret. J Am Vet Med Assoc 1982;181:820–2.

[21] Lucas A. Ferret emergency techniques. In: Lewington J, editor. Ferret husbandry, medicine and surgery. Edinburgh (UK): Butterworth Heinemann; 2002. p. 261–71.

[22] Carpenter J. Exotic animal formulary. 3rd edition. Missouri (MO): Elsevier Saunders; 2005. p. 466.

VETERINARY
CLINICS
Exotic Animal Practice

Vet Clin Exot Anim 11 (2008) 551–567

Rabbit Hematology

Kemba L. Marshall, DVM, DABVP–Avian

Summertree Animal and Bird Clinic, 12300 Inwood Road, Suite 102, Dallas, TX 75244, USA

Descending from the European wild rabbit, *Oryctolagus cuniculus*, there are more than 100 breeds of rabbits [1]. They differentiated in the mid-Eocene age [2]. The domestic rabbit was introduced by human beings into New Zealand and Australia, rapidly becoming the most prevalent wild mammal [2]. Rabbits, of the order Lagomorpha, are one the most common mammals found throughout the world. Hares and pikas are also in the order Lagomorpha. The European wild rabbit was not introduced to North America. Here, the native wild rabbit is *Sylvilagus floridanus* (cottontail) or *Sylvilagus bachmani* (brush rabbit). The North American jackrabbit (*Lepus californicus*) also represents the hare genus. The order Lagomorpha is characterized by peg teeth and the presence of a second pair of upper incisors [1].

Despite the vast number of rabbit breeds, information regarding rabbit hematology does not reflect the myriad of rabbits in laboratory animal medical facilities and also in private homes kept as companion animals. Hematology reference ranges draw heavily from the New Zealand white rabbit, the most common breed used in laboratory research (Table 1) [1]. Obvious limitations then include a uniform population of animals housed indoors in pathogen-free environments fed commercial pellets with temperature, lighting, and feeding cycles closely monitored and regulated. In contrast, a variety of companion animal rabbits are housed indoors and outdoors, consuming a wide variety of food items. Rabbits caged, eating commercial feed mixes and experiencing dental disease, have consistently lower packed cell volumes, red blood cell (RBC) counts, hemoglobin values, and lymphocyte counts than rabbits kept outside with increased exercise and natural diets [3]. Historically, in companion medicine, blood work submitted on rabbits was done when these animals were presented with illness. With wellness testing becoming the norm rather than the exception, reference laboratories now have the opportunity to include larger numbers of patients for the characterization of "normal values" in the reference range. The aim of

E-mail address: petagrees@yahoo.com

Table 1
Normal hematologic values in the domestic rabbit

Erythrocytes	$5.1–7.9 \times 10^6$ m^3
Hematocrit	33%–50%
Hemoglobin	10.0–17.4 g/dL
Mean corpuscular volume	57.8–66.5 μm^3
Mean corpuscular hemoglobin concentration	29%–37%
Platelets	$250–260 \times 10^6$ m^3
Leukocytes	$5.2–12.5 \times 10^6$ m^3
Heterophils	20%–75%
Lymphocytes	30%–85%
Monocytes	1%–4%
Eosinophils	1%–4%
Basophils	1%–7%

Data from Benson KG, Paul-Murphy J. Clinical pathology of the domestic rabbit: acquisition and interpretation of samples. Vet Clin North Am Exot Anim Pract 1999;2:539–51.

this article is to discuss normal hematopoiesis and infectious and metabolic diseases that specifically target the hemolymphatic system. Additionally, photographic representation of cell types is provided.

Restraint and phlebotomy

The jugular vein, lateral saphenous vein, femoral vein, cephalic vein, or marginal ear vein of rabbits is acceptable for venipuncture. Proper restraint is necessary, and a variety of methods can be used, including manual restraint, commercial rabbit restrainers, or even "cat bags." Rabbit restraint, similar to that used for cats, requires neck extension with the feet drawn vertically over the table's edge. Rabbits can also be wrapped in a towel in dorsal recumbency with the neck in rostral extension and held by the phlebotomist. In this method, the jugular vein is punctured craniocaudally. If the lateral saphenous vein is to be used, it is important to note its difficulty in rabbits that are fractious and have a tendency to kick. The rabbit is maintained in sternal recumbency, and the leg is held at the crus of the stifle for venous occlusion [4]. It is important to note that all rabbit restraint is done relative to the overall health status of the rabbit. Overly aggressive restraint, or even prolonged restraint in ill animals, can have devastating consequences. When subjected to severe stress, rabbits release high levels of catecholamines that can lead to cardiac arrest. The best venipuncturist should be used, and oxygen therapy should be readily available for any animal that becomes dyspneic. Additionally, rabbits may benefit from subcutaneous fluid therapy and time in a quiet isolated cage before venipuncture is attempted, especially if a rabbit seems to be stressed skittish, or dehydrated or has upper airway disease. For blood collection, 23- to 25-gauge needles can be used. In most domestic rabbits, a 1- or 3-cm^3 syringe is adequate for blood collection. Larger syringes may collapse the vein and should not be used on a regular basis. Blood clot formation is rapid at room temperature. To prevent blood clotting during venipuncture, a heparin flush may be used. Heparin is drawn into the needle and syringe and then immediately pushed back into the bottle of heparin. Excess heparin is removed by drawing air into the needle and syringe and then forcefully expelling the air and residual heparin. Heparin in small amounts prevents blood clotting without altering hematologic parameters [5].

Cell lines

Circulating cells are constantly replenished by the production and release of cells from the bone marrow. Common stem cells in the bone marrow are pluripotent in that they give rise to progenitor cells. These progenitor cells differentiate to the erythrocytic, granulocytic, megakaryocytic, and agranulocytic (monocytic and lymphocytic) lines. Ultimately, RBCs, white blood cells (WBCs), and platelets are released into circulation [6]. As erythrocytic and granulocytic precursors mature, the cell and nucleus decrease in size and there is a loss of nucleoli and condensation of nuclear chromatin.

Oxygen transport and erythrocytes

Among mammals, the hemoglobin content and packed cell volume are relatively constant. The total erythrocyte count and mean cell size vary [7]. Rabbit blood cells vary in diameter (5.0–7.8 μm), and this anisocytosis is not clinically significant (Fig. 1) [8]. The hemoglobin-to-surface distance during gas exchange is reduced, whereas cell plasticity is increased to facilitate movement through blood vessels. The small, anucleate, round, and biconcave nature of rabbit erythrocytes aids in the transportation of oxygen to tissues [7]. The estimated total blood volume in rabbits is between 4.5%

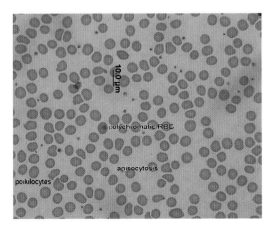

Fig. 1. Mild anisocytosis, poikilocytosis, and polychromasia in a rabbit.

and 8.1% of total body weight or approximately 57 to 78 mL/kg of body weight [4]. Alternatively, measurements of blood volume are correlated with lean body weight or body surface area [9]. New Zealand white rabbits have been safely bled at rates of 6 to 8 mL/kg/wk [4].

Rabbit erythrocytes have an estimated life span of 50 days and measure 6.5 to 7.5 μm in diameter; polychromasia is seen commonly because of the short half-life of erythrocytes (see Fig. 1). Polychromatic erythrocytes (reticulocytes) are young erythrocytes that have been released into circulation early and account for 2% to 5% of the population (see Fig. 1) [1,7,10]. Reticulocytes are larger and more basophilic than mature erythrocytes. A small number of damaged or aged RBCs are removed from circulation continually by hemopoietic tissues and splenic macrophages [7].

Chronic blood loss resulting in anemia has shown that the erythropoietic capacity of bone marrow can compensate for chronic blood losses of up to 10 to 12 mL/kg of body weight [10]. Causes of anemias in rabbits include lead toxicosis, uterine adenocarcinoma, endometrial hyperplasia, and chronic metabolic disease (otitis media, dental disease with or without abscesses, pneumonia, pododermatitis, mastitis, endometritis and pyometra, renal disease, and osteomyelitis) [5].

Anemia is the reduction in the total number of hemoglobin-bearing erythrocytes leading to deficient oxygen transport [7]. Abnormal RBC loss that is not sufficiently compensated for by normal erythropoiesis and decreased blood cell production that cannot provide sufficient replacement of RBCs are the two most common causes of anemia [11]. The destruction of RBCs characterizes hemolytic anemia. Erythrocyte loss by means of hemorrhage defines hemorrhagic anemia, and hypoplastic anemia is found secondary to decreased erythrocyte production [7]. Nonregenerative hypoplastic anemias are also hypochromic because of chronic iron deficiencies. Anemias of chronic disease occur secondary to decreased renal erythropoietin production and decreased hemoglobin levels as bone marrow production of RBCs is diminished. It is this hypochromasia that causes poor tissue perfusion. For this reason Oxyglobin (Biopure, Cambridge, Massachusetts) may be administered to increase hemoglobin concentrations. This product, when available, has been shown to be beneficial when used at a slow intravenous push at a dose of 2 to 5 mg/kg [12].

To the author's knowledge, there are no recognized rabbit blood groups. Cross-matching should be used before blood transfusions. In the author's experience, blood transfusions are well tolerated.

Anemias are regenerative or nonregenerative. Insufficient RBC production by bone marrow results in circulating RBCs that are normal in appearance [11]. Extramedullary hematopoiesis occurs in sites that include the liver and spleen. Appropriate bone marrow response to anemia leads to increased production of RBCs with potentially premature release of RBCs into the circulation. Polychromasia is seen with blood loss and blood destruction anemias but is not present in aplastic anemia or in anemias caused by erythroid hypoplasia [7]. These polychromatic cells are larger than mature RBCs and have a blue to reddish-blue cytoplasm. Polychromatophils may not have the classic discoid shape of mature RBCs but can have membranous infoldings and outfoldings that seem to be target or bar cells [11]. Polychromatophils have intracellular reticulum; this is irregular clumping of ribosomal RNA and organelles. Polychromatic erythrocytes on Romanowsky-stained blood films are equivalent to reticulocytes on new methylene blue and other vital stains [7]. Howell-Jolly bodies, anisocytosis, basophilic stippling, and nucleated RBCs can also be seen with regenerative anemias (Fig. 2, basophilic RBC with Howell-Jolly body). Howell-Jolly bodies are dark-blue inclusions in the cytoplasm of the erythrocyte. Variably sized, these small round inclusions are nuclear remnants that have not been completely removed by macrophages during accelerated hematopoiesis (Fig. 3, nucleated RBC and platelets) [7]. Splenic macrophages have a significant role in removing these nuclear remnants [11]. A high percentage of circulating nucleated RBCs without significant polychromasia indicates bone marrow damage [7]. Bone marrow aspirates are indicated to evaluate pancytopenia, nonregenerative anemia, leukemia, and gammopathy. Bone marrow aspiration is frequently performed along the proximal femur and requires general anesthesia; local anesthetic is recommended for the overlying subcutis and periosteum. The area of the proximal femur is surgically prepared, and a small incision is made over the proximal femur. A spinal-shaped needle is introduced into the intertrochanteric fossa through the cortical bone into the intermedullary space using a clockwise-counterclockwise rotation. Once in place, the stylet is removed and a syringe is attached to the

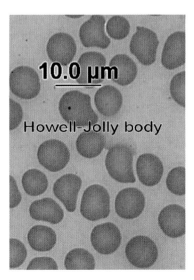

Fig. 2. Basophilic RBC with Howell-Jolly body.

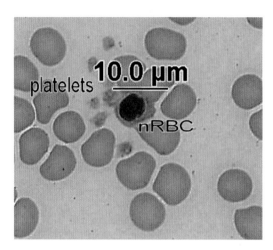

Fig. 3. Nucleated red blood cell (nRBC) and platelets.

hub. Negative pressure is applied until the marrow appears beyond the hub. Care should be taken to avoid excess pressure, which can lead to peripheral blood contamination [7].

Clinical presentations of selected diseases

Commonly, ill rabbits are presented for nonspecific signs, including weight loss, anorexia, dehydration, and depression. A thorough physical examination and complete anamnesis are essential in generating the differential diagnoses. Animals that are allowed free roam of the house and are known to chew baseboards or dig at carpets should be considered potentially exposed to lead toxicosis. With the requirements of lead-free paints in newer homes, this is not a common finding in the author's practice. Animals that are allowed to chew cords and whose owners leave coins and other foreign objects around the home are seen more frequently. A complete minimum database, including radiographs can help to determine where any metallic foreign bodies are located and if medical or surgical therapy is required. Chelation (calcium ethylenediaminetetraacetic acid [EDTA] administered subcutaneously at a dosage of 27 mg/kg every 6–12 hours) [13] and fluid therapy may be sufficient to facilitate passage of objects situated in the large intestine. Material in the stomach or proximal small intestine can be surgically removed with complete resolution of clinical signs.

Uterine adenocarcinomas are prevalent in the intact doe and are a major talking point to convince owners to spay their female rabbits. Hematuria can be seen with uterine adenocarcinomas and endometrial hyperplasia. It is important to note that rabbits can have pigmented urine normally, and in-house urine dipsticks are useful to delineate true hematuria. Pronounced anemia in an intact doe can suggest uterine pathologic findings. Histopathologic examination is recommended to differentiate adenocarcinoma from endometrial hyperplasia. In the absence of profound anemia and metastasis, ovariohysterectomy procedures are curative.

Rabbits that present for "going off feed" often have dental disease. A thorough dental examination must include examination of incisors and cheek teeth. Sedation may be required to facilitate the dental examination. Rabbits whose complete blood cell count and serum chemistry panels are within normal ranges are anesthetized for teeth trimming or floating. This procedure can be done quickly using a high-speed dental handpiece and appropriate dental equipment, including cheek dilators, tongue protectors, and mouth gags [14]. Endoscopic images of the mouth before and after the dental procedure help clients to understand its significance. In cases in which an oral abscess is present, bacterial cultures should be taken to direct the clinician on appropriate antibiotic therapy. Abscesses, which are often walled off in an isolated cavity, can be seen with peripheral leukocytosis and heterophilia because the bone marrow response to infection is greater than the consumption in a closed-cavity abscess [8]. A variety of antibiotics can be used in the rabbit, including trimethoprim sulfa administered orally at a dosage of 30 mg/kg every 12 hours or baytril administered orally, subcutaneously, or intramuscularly at a dosage of 5 to 10 mg/kg every 12 hours [13]. The author routinely gives probiotics in the form of Bene-Bac (Pet-Ag, Hampshire, Illinois), yogurt with live active cultures, or powdered acidophilus to prevent dysbiosis. Owners should also be informed that because rabbits' teeth grow continuously, rabbits with malocclusions need to be seen routinely for dental examinations and teeth floating when necessary. This is not a condition that we expect to cure but rather manage. The gastric stasis and anorexia that often accompany malocclusion can be treated with intravenous or subcutaneous crystalloid fluid therapy along with gastric motility agents and supportive diets. In the author's practice, cisapride (0.5 mg/kg administered orally every 8–12 hours) [12] and Oxbow critical care for herbivores (Oxbow Animal Health, Murdock, Nebraska) (10–12 mL/kg every 8–12 hours) have yielded proven results.

Bacterial infections secondary to *Pasteurella multocida* are widespread in the companion rabbit population. The characteristic white nasal discharge, along with respiratory congestion, is a hallmark of "snuffles." *Pasteurella* infections seem to affect older rabbits more frequently. Disseminated infections have been seen clinically as otitis media, pneumonia, pododermatitis, mastitis, and osteomyelitis. Long-term antibiotic therapy may be indicated because of the chronic nature of *Pasteurella* infections. In addition to oral antibiotics, benzathine penicillin G can be given intramuscularly every 5 to 7 days at a rate of 42,000 to 60,000 IU/kg [13]. As a general rule, the author uses lactobacillus or acidophilus supplements while rabbits are on antibiotics to prevent dysbiosis. Rather than develop a leukocytosis in response to bacterial disease, rabbits have an increase in the absolute heterophil concentration and a concurrent decrease in the absolute lymphocyte concentration [8]. Although *P multocida* is a common pathogen in rabbits, bacterial culture and sensitivity tests are always indicated to direct the clinician properly toward the causative bacterial pathogen and appropriate antibiotic therapy.

Rabbit calicivirus disease

In 1984, angora rabbits that had been imported to China from Europe were affected with a strain of viral hemorrhagic disease that killed 14 million domesticated rabbits within 9 months. Outbreaks were reported in 40 countries, and by the late 1990s, rabbit hemorrhagic disease was endemic in populations of wild rabbits in New Zealand, Australia, and Europe. Although extremely contagious and often fatal, this viral disease only affects rabbits of the species *O cuniculus*. Cottontails (*S floridanus*), black-tailed jackrabbits (*L californicus*), European brown hares (*Lepus europaeus*), and snowshoe hares (*Lepus americanus*) are not affected by rabbit hemorrhagic disease virus (RHDV) [13]. Limited outbreaks have occurred in Iowa (2000), Utah (2001), Illinois (2001), New York (2001), and Indiana (2005) but have been eradicated in each case. RHDV may have originated from avirulent caliciviruses circulating in wild European populations [15].

Viral transmission is through oral, nasal, or conjunctival routes by means of infected animals and fomites by virulent and avirulent modes of infection. Urine, feces, respiratory secretions, and all excretions are thought to contain virus [16]. RHDV can be acquired by exposure to an infected carcass or hair. The causative virus is resistant to inactivation when protected by organic material and may persist in chilled or frozen rabbit meat for months [17]. The virus can survive for 7.5 months in tissue suspensions stored at 4°C (39°F) and for more than 3 months at 20°C (68°F) in dried organ homogenates [17]. Long-term, persistent, and latent infections have all been recognized.

Young rabbits are resistant to disease. Symptoms typically occur after a 1- to 3-day incubation period in animals that are more than 8 weeks old. Infected rabbits can die within 12 to 36 hours after becoming febrile. When present, acute signs of illness include dullness, anorexia, palpebral conjunctival congestion, respiratory signs, and neurologic deficits. Paddling, opisthotonos, excitement, and incoordination can be seen. Disseminated intravascular coagulation (DIC) and a blood-stained frothy nasal discharge are seen terminally. The morbidity rate ranges from 30% to 100%, and the mortality rate ranges from 40% to 100%. The most consistent postmortem lesions are hepatic necrosis and splenomegaly [18]. The virus can be identified with the reverse transcription polymerase chain reaction (RT-PCR), immunoblotting, or ELISA. Rabbit hemorrhagic disease must be reported to state authorities [19,20] immediately on diagnosis or suspicion of disease. To date, treatment of this disease has been unrewarding. Because this is a reportable disease, it may be up to the discretion of state authorities to determine if treatment can be attempted or if test-and-slaughter protocols are to be enforced.

Granulocytes and agranulocytes

Leukocytes in the peripheral blood are granular or agranular. Granular leukocytes contain a lobed nucleus and, based on the staining characteristics of cytoplasmic granules, are grouped as neutrophils, eosinophils, or basophils [7,21]. Possessing acidophilic cytoplasmic granules, heterophils are the counterpart of the neutrophils and measure 9 to 15 μm in diameter [1,10,21]. The overall color of the rabbit heterophil cytoplasm is almost colorless but varies according to the proportion of large and small granules present. The heterophil stains pink because of the number of small acidophilic granules within the cytoplasm [9]. In comparison to these primary granules, secondary granules are dark pink to red. Smaller granules stain pink, giving a pink tinge to the cytoplasm, whereas large pink-red granules result in a reddish cytoplasmic hue [7]. These two populations of granules arise from two separate sites on the Golgi apparatus and have differing functions. The smaller pink granules are the compliment of secondary specific granules in other mammals. The smaller granules are formed during the myelocyte stage of development; as the majority of cytoplasmic granules in mature heterophils, they account for 80% to 90% of the population [4]. Smaller granules have been shown to contain peroxidase, alkaline phosphatase, lipase, and other antibacterial properties [4]. The larger darker staining granules are formed early in the maturation of the heterophil and are seen initially in the progranulocyte stage. These granules correspond to the primary azurophilic granules of the canine neutrophil [4]. For this reason, rabbit neutrophils are also called heterophils, pseudoeosinophils, acidophils, or amphophils (Fig. 4, rabbit normal heterophil and toxic heterophil) [4,22]. Currently, the quantification of different levels of

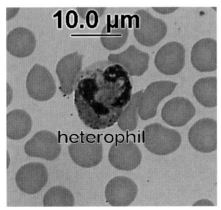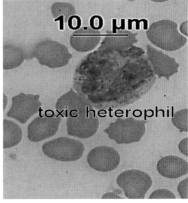

Fig. 4. Rabbit normal heterophil and toxic heterophil.

antibacterial properties in small versus large granules is not known [8]. Heterophils have phagocytic capabilities and tend to increase in the face of inflammation, specifically when caused by bacterial organisms [7]. Heterophils migrate to tissue sites of inflammation because of chemical attraction, participating in phagocytosis of pathogens and foreign material. Lysosomal granules present in the cytoplasm fuse with phagosomes to kill infectious organisms after phagocytosis. Material in the phagosomes is then degraded by enzymatic digestion [7].

Toxic changes to heterophils are morphologic descriptives, seen with premature release of heterophils from the bone marrow. In response to inflammatory diseases that result in increased production of heterophils, organelles are retained. Retention of ribosomes and other organelles leads to cytoplasmic basophilia and vacuolation [7].

Excitement in animals not accustomed to handling leads to epinephrine release. Rabbits normally have more circulating lymphocytes than heterophils [8], and in response to acute stress, a mature heterophilia and relative lymphopenia result. Epinephrine causes heterophils to leave the marginating pool and enter the circulating pool as heart rate and blood flow increase. This tends to result in a heterophilia but may result in a lymphocytosis. Similarly, when exogenous adrenaline was administered to rabbits, lymphocytes were redistributed from the spleen and bone marrow to peripheral blood, lungs, and liver [23].

Heterophils found in the peripheral blood are in the circulating or marginating pool. Occurring in large blood vessels, the circulating pool consists of heterophils that do not interact with the endothelial vessel wall. During venipuncture, blood is sampled from the circulating pool. The marginating pool consists of heterophils that interact with the endothelium of small blood vessels and capillaries [7]. A heterophilia with a left shift is indicative of inflammatory disease. Rabbits do not typically develop a leukocytosis when bacterial infections are present but rather increase the absolute heterophil concentration and decrease the absolute lymphocyte concentration. It is noteworthy that the relative heterophilia and lymphopenia may not alter the total WBC count [8].

Mononuclear leukocytes lack cytoplasmic granules and have a nonlobed nucleus. They are classified as monocytes or lymphocytes (Fig. 5, monocyte with intermediate lymphocyte). When they are small, lymphocytes measure 7 to 10 μm, and large lymphocytes measure 10 to 15 μm (Fig. 6, mature versus intermediate lymphocyte) [1]. Lymphocytes are the predominant WBC in peripheral rabbit circulation (Fig. 7, rabbit lymphocyte) [1,7,8,10]. Lymphocytes and monocytes appear the same as in other mammals [7,24] Distributed in blood, bone marrow, lymph nodes, gut-associated lymphoid tissue, and the spleen, lymphocytes are responsible for certain immunologic responses (Fig. 8, mature lymphocyte and nucleated RBC with platelet) [4,7,8]. Rabbit monocytes are the largest of the leukocytes. Monocytes have an amoeboid nucleus, diffuse nuclear chromatin, and

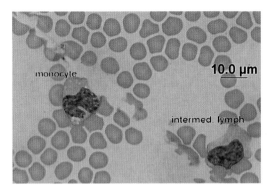

Fig. 5. Monocyte with intermediate (intermed.) lymphocyte.

blue cytoplasm, and they lack a nonstaining perinuclear area (Fig. 9, rabbit monocyte; Fig. 10, rabbit monocyte with platelets). Large dark-red granules in monocyte cytoplasm have been associated with toxicity. These criteria differentiate monocytes from lymphocytes [4].

Leukemias are infrequently reported in rabbit medicine. A small number of cases of lymphoblastic leukemia have been documented [25–27]. WBC counts with leukemia range from 30,000 to greater than 100,000; prognosis has been poor because lymphadenopathy and organomegaly have been present at the time of diagnosis in each case. Uniform lymphocyte populations have been seen on peripheral blood smears, bone marrow cytology, lymph node, and hepatic and splenic aspirates (Fig. 11, lymphocytic leukemia in a rabbit peripheral blood smear). Greatly enlarged kidneys, hepatomegaly with uniformly distributed white foci, splenomegaly, and lymphadenopathy form a complex that occurs frequently. This quartet pattern has been described as pathognomonic for lymphosarcoma in the rabbit [25,28].

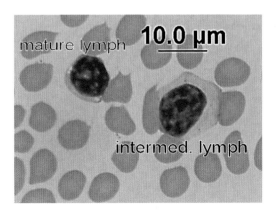

Fig. 6. Mature versus intermediate (intermed.) lymphocyte.

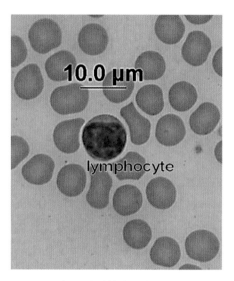

Fig. 7. Rabbit lymphocyte.

Eosinophils stain a dull pink orange with hematology stains and are 12 to 16 μm in diameter. The acidophilic granules can dominate the cytoplasm, filling it entirely [4]. Although mainly involved in the inactivation of histamine or histamine-like toxic materials, eosinophils are capable of phagocytosis (Fig. 12, rabbit eosinophil) [29]. Eosinophils are important in allergic response and are elevated in certain chronic diseases. These diseases involve

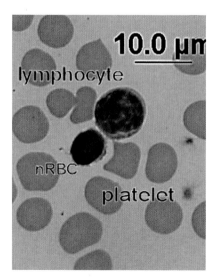

Fig. 8. Mature lymphocyte and nucleated red blood cell (nRBC) with platelet.

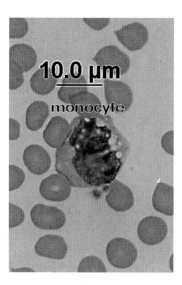

Fig. 9. Rabbit monocyte.

the skin, lungs, gastrointestinal tract, and uterus, all of which have high percentages of mast cells. Eosinophilia is also seen in parasitic diseases with skin migration [7,8]. Low eosinophil counts or counts of 0 are not uncommon in rabbits [8].

Basophils may be up to 30% of the population, and rabbits are the only laboratory species with peripheral basophils seen normally in circulation

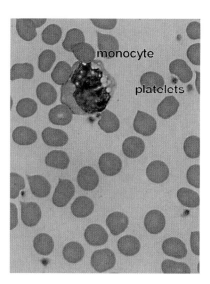

Fig. 10. Rabbit monocyte with platelets.

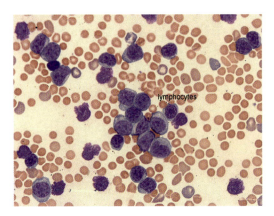

Fig. 11. Lymphocytic leukemia in rabbit peripheral blood smear.

(Fig. 13, rabbit basophil) [4,30]. Similar in size to heterophils the basophil nucleus can be obscured by purple and black metachromic granules (Fig. 14, rabbit basophil) [4,7,8].

Platelets are defined as cytoplasmic fragments that arise from megakaryocytes within bone marrow and participate in hemostasis [2,7]. Platelets are disks of cytoplasm that contain cytoplasmic organelles. Platelets are the initial hemostatic plug in the clotting process. As such, they work to prevent hemorrhage after vascular injury to the microcirculation. Often, they appear as clumps on blood films [7]. Platelets that are larger than erythrocytes are macro- or megaplatelets and have been released early from bone marrow (Fig. 15, large and small platelets) [21].

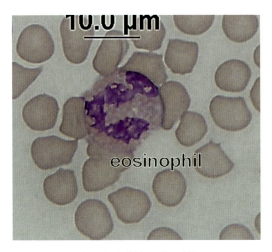

Fig. 12. Rabbit eosinophil.

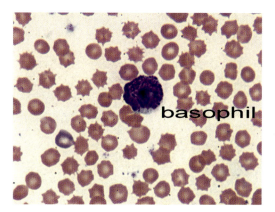

Fig. 13. Rabbit basophil.

Hemostatic factors

There is a dearth of information regarding hemostatic factors in normal rabbits. One study involving 12 New Zealand white rabbits measured various coagulation tests and should be referenced for additional information [2]. Because it relates to RHDV, DIC has been reported in conjunction with prolonged prothrombin time (PT) and partial thromboplastin time (PTT) [30,31].

Summary

Rabbit hematology is not drastically different from that of other mammals. Using laboratory animal medicine as an established resource, companion animal veterinarians have access to many physiologic and basic science studies that we can now merge with our clinical impressions. The study of

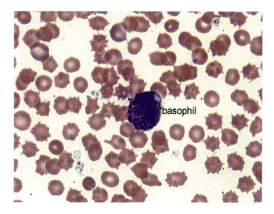

Fig. 14. Rabbit basophil.

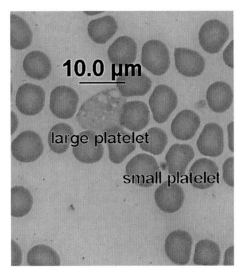

Fig. 15. Large and small platelets.

rabbit hematology is in its infancy in companion animal medicine but is in its adolescence in laboratory medicine. By working with reference laboratories, companion animal veterinarians are poised to accelerate our knowledge of the normal rabbit rapidly. In doing so, veterinarians are also poised to advance human medicine as we strive to explore further, and thus improve, the human-animal bond.

Acknowledgments

The author is indebted to Dr. Vicky Joseph, DABVP (Avian) of Idexx Laboratories, Sacramento, CA and Karl Snyder, MT (ASCP) of the University of Tennessee College of Veterinary Medicine clinical pathology department for generous donation of photographs.

References

[1] Wilber JL. Pathology of the rabbit. Washington, DC: Department of Veterinary Pathology, Armed Forces Institute of Pathology; August 1999,. Available at: http://www.afip.org/vetpath/POLA/99/PATHOLOGY_OF_THE_RABBIT-Wilber.htm. Accessed December 8, 2007.

[2] Lewis JH. Rabbits. In: Lewis JH, editor. Comparative hemostasis in vertebrates. New York: Springer Publishing; 1996. p. 182–93.

[3] Harcourt-Brown FM, Baker SJ. Parathyroid hormone, hematological and biochemical parameters in relation to dental disease and husbandry in pet rabbits. J Small Anim Prac 2001;42:130–6.

[4] Benson KG, Paul-Murphy J. Clinical pathology of the domestic rabbit: acquisition and interpretation of samples. Veterinary Clin North Am Exot Anim Pract 1999;2(3):539–51.

[5] Melillo A. Rabbit clinical pathology. J Exot Pet Med 2007;16(3):135–45.

[6] Hematopoiesis. In: Reagan WJ, Sanders TG, DeNicola DB, editors. Veterinary hematology: atlas of common domestic species. Iowa State University Press; 1998. p. 3–11.

[7] Campbell TW, Ellis CK. Avian and exotic animal hematology and cytology. 3rd edition. Ames (IA): Blackwell Publishing; 2007.

[8] Clinical pathology. In: Harcourt-Brown F, editor. Textbook of rabbit medicine. London: Elsevier Science; 2002. p. 140–64.

[9] Moore DM. Hematology of rabbits. In: Feldman BF, editor. Schalm's veterinary hematology. 5th edition. Ames (IA): Blackwell Publishing; 2000.

[10] Delaney-Johnson CA. Small mammal hematology. AAV Conf Proc 1998 Session #200 p 85–6.

[11] Variations in red blood cell morphology. In: Reagan WJ, Sanders TG, DeNicola DB, editors. Veterinary hematology: atlas of common domestic species. Iowa State University Press; 1998. p. 17–24.

[12] Lichtenberber M. Emergency care of rabbits and pocket pets. Western Veterinary Conf Proc 2002.

[13] Carpenter JW. Rabbits. In: Exotic animal formulary. 3rd edition. Philadelphia: Elsevier Saunders; 2005. p. 411–44.

[14] Universal Surgical Instruments. Available at: www.universalsurgical.com. Accessed December 8, 2007.

[15] Donnelly T. Emerging viral diseases of rabbits and rodents: viral hemorrhagic disease and hantavirus infection. Sem Avian Exot Pet Med 1995;4:83–91.

[16] Campagnolo ER, Ernst MJ, Berninger ML, et al. Outbreak of rabbit hemorrhagic disease in domestic lagomorphs. J Am Vet Med Assoc 2004;223:1151–5, 1128.

[17] White PJ, Trout RC, Moss SR, et al. Epidemiology of rabbit hemorrhagic disease virus in the United Kingdom: evidence for seasonal transmission. Epidemiol Infect 2004;132:555–67.

[18] McColl KA, Morrissy CJ, Collins BJ, et al. Persistence of rabbit hemorrhagic disease in decomposing rabbit carcasses. Aust Vet J 2002;80:298–9.

[19] Available at: http://www.aphis.usda.gov/vs/sregs/official.html. Accessed December 8, 2007.

[20] Available at: http://www.aphis.usda.gov/vs/area_offices.htm. Accessed December 8, 2007.

[21] Chasey D. Rabbit hemorrhagic disease: the new scourge of Oryctolagus cuniculus. Lab Anim 1997;31:33–44.

[22] Normal white blood cell morphology. In: Reagan WJ, Sanders TG, DeNicola DB, editors. Veterinary hematology: atlas of common domestic species. Iowa State University Press; 1998. p. 29–35.

[23] Sanderson JH, Philips CE. Rabbits. In: An atlas of laboratory haematology. New York: Oxford University Press; 1982.

[24] Toft P, Tonnesen E, Svendsen P, et al. Redistribution of lymphocytes after cortisol administration [abstract]. APMIS 1992;100:154–8.

[25] Campbell TW. Basics of cytology and fluid cytology. Vet Clin North Am Exot Anim Pract 2007;10(1):1–10.

[26] Finnie JW, Bostock WDE, Walden NB. Lymphoblastic leukaemia in a rabbit: a case report. Lab Anim 1980;14:49–51.

[27] Cloyd GG, Johnson GR. Lymphosarcoma with lymphoblastic leukemia in a New Zealand white rabbit. Lab Anim Sci 1978;28(1):66–9.

[28] Huston SM, Quesenberry KE. Cardiovascular and lymphoproliferative diseases. In: Ferrets, rabbits and rodents: clinical medicine and surgery. 2nd edition. Saunders publishing; 2003. p. 211–20.

[29] Weisbroth SH, Flatt RE, Kraus AL. The biology of the laboratory rabbit. Academic Press; 1974.

[30] Kerr M. Veterinary laboratory medicine: clinical biochemistry and haematology. Ames (IA): Blackwell Scientific publications; 1989.

[31] Plassiat G, Geulfi JF, Ganiere JP, et al. Hematological parameters and visceral lesions relationships in rabbit viral hemorrhagic disease. J Vet Med B 1992;39:443–53.

ELSEVIER
SAUNDERS

Vet Clin Exot Anim 11 (2008) 569–582

VETERINARY
CLINICS
Exotic Animal Practice

Normal Hematology and Hematologic Disorders in Potbellied Pigs

Sherrie G. Clark, DVM, MS, PhD, DACT,
Natalie Coffer, BVetMed, MS, DACVIM*

*Department of Veterinary Clinical Medicine, University of Illinois at Urbana-Champaign,
1008 West Hazelwood Drive, Urbana, IL 61802, USA*

The popularity of potbellied pigs as pets has seemed to remain at a constant level over the past 20 years [1–3]. They became popular as pets in the United States in the middle to late 1980s. Many small animal veterinary practitioners see potbellied pigs but believe that they lack the knowledge and information to work with them properly. General reference information on their health and care is provided on Web sites from breeders and owners of these pigs and their experiences. There is little information for veterinarians on case management and specific disorders of the hematologic system. Investigations to characterize potbellied pig hematology specifically are warranted. Most of the resources available have details on preventative care and emergency management of potbellied pigs [1–7].

Routine laboratory analysis and hemograms are not generally performed in miniature pigs. According to many sources, the hemograms of potbellied pigs and other miniature swine do not vary significantly from those of domestic swine [8–11]. Therefore, interpretation of laboratory results and other hematologic studies are performed in the same manner as with domestic pigs.

Blood sampling

This procedure is generally difficult in domestic swine because of inaccessibility of good veins and arteries [1,12–15]. In potbellied pigs, it becomes more difficult because of their shorter stature and smaller vessel size in addition to varying size of the animal and the ability to restrain it adequately for the procedure. Handling and proper restraint become extremely important

---

* Corresponding author.
E-mail address: ncoffer@uiuc.edu (N. Coffer).

when attempting to perform any venipuncture because there must be regard for safety of all participants and the animal. Obviously, the least amount of restraint necessary to obtain the sample is the best choice. With animals that are handled regularly, minimal restraint may be needed. Others, however, may need to be sedated to accomplish the goals. Many sources [3–5] have discussed chemical restraint of potbellied pigs and decided that gas anesthesia is overall the safest. It allows animals to experience a procedure without struggling, and they take this method of sedation with relative ease, especially if using a mask to administer the anesthetic [5]. There are various combinations of sedation and anesthetic agents that have been successfully used to sedate potbellied pigs [1,2,4]. Most of them involve a mixture of a dissociative anesthetic (ketamine), an α_2-adrenergic agonist (xylazine or medetomidine), an α_2-adrenergic antagonist (atipamezole), and benzodiazepines (midazolam) [16]. There are no reports of the use of any of these combinations having an adverse affect on the hematology of the pig; the elimination of stress is the key to having interpretable blood results.

Various sites have been accessed for blood collection and include the auricular veins, anterior vena cava, jugular vein, cephalic vein, orbital sinus, cranial superficial epigastric vein, and coccygeal vein [2–4,17,18]. For most hematologic parameters, collection of samples in ethylenediaminetetraacetic acid (EDTA) anticoagulant is preferred [10]. There are few artifacts observed when interpreting the hemogram of potbellied pigs, and they are discussed later in this article in the section on erythrocytes.

Jugular vein

This is the most common site of blood collection from pigs of any breed. Depending on the size of the pig, it is restrained using a snare around its snout or held in dorsal recumbency with its front legs pulled caudally. In the authors' experience, few potbellied pigs tolerate the use of a snare, but a light rope has been used to stabilize depressed or lethargic patients for acquisition of the blood sample. This was accomplished with a potbellied pig that weighed more than 100 lb and would normally not be the wisest method of restraint. It is important that the neck of the animal be held as straight as possible and be raised up when held manually or held straight and in full contact with the ground when held in dorsal recumbency. Most potbellied pigs can be restrained in dorsal recumbency if sedated. If the animal has been handled extensively, a small pig (<30 lb) may be manually held in a dorsal position.

In the standing position, "the jugular groove is traced to its caudal limit just anterior to the thoracic inlet. The needle (18–20 gauge, 1.5 inch) is inserted in the jugular groove approximately 5 cm cranial to the thoracic inlet, depending on the size of the pig, so that a perpendicular angle is formed between the needle and the ventral surface of the extended neck. The needle is directed caudodorsally and slightly medially" (Fig. 1) [18]. Care is taken to insert the needle smoothly and with minimal redirection, because the

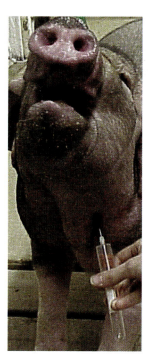

Fig. 1. Anatomic location of obtaining a blood sample from the jugular vein of a miniature pig (Meishan pig is shown in this figure).

incidence of hematoma formation can increase. Pig blood tends to clot readily; therefore, the formation of a hematoma is likely.

Anterior vena cava

Obtaining a blood sample from this anatomic location can be even more difficult in potbellied pigs because there is more subcutaneous fat than in domestic swine, but it is similar to obtaining blood from the jugular vein. The needle size varies with the size of the pig, and the length may need to be increased if there is a significant amount of fat in this region. Knowledge of the anatomy is crucial when performing this technique, and other sites are preferred because there is the potential to puncture the vagus nerve and result in dyspnea, cyanosis, and convulsions [18].

Auricular veins

Auricular veins are best visualized by placing a tourniquet at the base of the ear or wiping them with isopropyl alcohol. Venipuncture is performed with a winged catheter (19–21 gauge butterfly catheter) or a small needle (23–25 gauge, 0.75–1 inch) attached to a syringe, because a Vacutainer (BD, Franklin Lakes, New Jersey) collection usually results in collapse of the vein (Fig. 2) [17]. These veins are quite small, and hematomas commonly result during venipuncture. These vessels can be difficult to visualize when the skin of the pig is darkly pigmented. Additionally, the size of the ears of potbellied pigs is much smaller than that of domestic pigs and can make this technique more challenging.

Orbital venous sinus

For this procedure, large pigs are restrained by snare and smaller ones are held manually, with care to restrain the snout securely. Because this can be a slow method of collection of a blood sample, light sedation may be preferred. A needle (16–20 gauge for pigs ranging from 40–150 lb) is placed at the medial canthus of the eye just inside the nictitating membrane and advanced medially and slightly anteroventrally until it punctures the venous sinus. Blood is allowed to drip out of the needle and is collected in an open-topped tube [18,19]. Only small amounts of blood (3–5 mL) are generally collected with this method. The authors do not have personal experience with this method of blood collection because it is not commonly used. There are other sites discussed in this article that are preferred and yield a sample of good quality and quantity. Additionally, there can be some complications with induction of stress on the animal, postcollection hemorrhage, and pressure on the globe [18]. If the authors only need a small amount of blood for measurement of a packed cell volume (PCV) or total serum protein, a sample would be obtained from the auricular vein.

Cranial superficial epigastric vein

This vein is present in all swine, is more easily accessed in boars and barrows than in female swine, and has been recently described as a method of blood collection [12,13]. The vein courses along the ventral portion of the abdomen and lies dorsolateral to the mammary chain. Direct pressure is

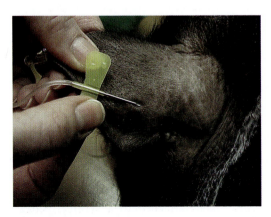

Fig. 2. Catheterization of the auricular vein using a butterfly catheter in a potbellied pig.

applied to the vessel for ease of visualization, and venipuncture is performed with various sizes of needles, ranging from 22 gauge up to 18 gauge, depending on the vessel size. The vessel is generally considered to be superficial and depends on the amount of fat deposition in this area. Care needs to be taken not to enter the peritoneal cavity when performing this technique [17] When performing this technique, the animal needs to be properly restrained or under general anesthesia [4]. As with any of the techniques described for obtaining blood samples from pigs, hematoma formation is always a potential complication. In this region, however, the hematoma would likely be small and not cause any major discomfort to the pig.

Coccygeal vessels

These vessels are only accessed in mature potbellied pigs whose tails have not been docked. Proper restraint is of the utmost importance [4]. The authors would suggest that the animal be sedated before attempting this method of blood collection. The technique is described similar to obtaining a sample from a cow in that the tail is held vertically and the needle is directed toward the point of junction of the tail with the body [14]. The authors have no experience with this method and would select the auricular or jugular vein before attempting to obtain a sample from this site.

Bone marrow collection

The procedure for bone marrow collection is performed on animals with "unexplained hematologic abnormalities when a diagnosis cannot be established based on examination of the blood" [11]. With regard to miniature swine, this may be the case with nonregenerative anemia or neoplastic marrow disease [10].

There are not many described sites for bone marrow aspiration in potbellied pigs, but those used with the dog most likely work in smaller (<100 lb) pigs [10,11]. The most common sites of bone marrow collection in dogs are the proximal end of the femur at the trochanteric fossa, the iliac crest, and the proximal humerus. If the animal is larger than 100 lb, other sites, such as the sternum or ribs, may be used, because there may be too much fat covering these regions to reach the bone adequately with the usual instrumentation [11]. General anesthesia would be the authors' recommendation for obtaining a bone marrow sample from a potbellied pig. The sample can be obtained using a biopsy needle. The skin is prepared as for a normal surgical preparation. The needle is introduced through the skin and pushed through until it reaches cortical bone. The needle should then be rotated until it is firmly seated into the bone and advanced a few millimeters. Once the placement is set, the stylet is removed, a syringe is attached, and negative pressure is applied until marrow is seen in the syringe. The marrow should be placed in an EDTA tube or on a slide immediately to prevent clotting [11].

In normal porcine bone marrow sample, lymphocytes represent 4.2% to 30% of cells and less than 1% of the remaining cells are plasma cells [20]. The myeloid-to-erythroid (M/E) ratios range from 1 to 3 [10,20]. A newborn piglet has little fat in the bone marrow and a large number of cells when it is born. The proportions of these substances reverse as the piglet gets older and matures [20].

Effects on the normal hemogram

Once a sample is acquired, it should be placed into the proper tube for analysis. It should also be noted that porcine red blood cells need to be handled carefully because they are highly susceptible to hemolysis. It is the authors' experience that porcine blood clots quickly and some hemolysis should be expected. Another complication that may occur with interpretation of the hemogram (Table 1) is that normal pigs develop a stress leukogram during collection of the blood sample [10,20]. Because of the excitability caused during restraint of pigs for blood collection procedures, these animals become stressed and have a resultant physiologic leukocytosis [4,8]. Normal minipigs have total leukocyte concentrations as great as 22,000 cells/μL as a result of excitement [8].

Erythrocytes

The red blood cells of miniature swine are similar to those of domestic pigs and have an average diameter of 6.0 μm [9,10] and an average life span of 86 days [21]. Erythrocyte spiculation, characterized by sharp pointed projections from the cells, is common in the blood films of normal minipigs. In healthy pigs, rouleaux can be a normal finding. In adult pigs, anisocytosis (variation in erythrocyte size) has been observed but is more commonly seen in young piglets [8–11].

Table 1
Normal blood values for the pig

	Range	Means		Range	Means
Erythrocytes ($\times 10^6$/μL)	5.0–8.0	6.5	Leukocytes/μL	11,000–22,000	16,000
Hemoglobin (g/dL)	10.0–16.0	13.0	Percentage distribution	—	—
PCV (%)	32–50	42.0	Neutrophil (band)	0–4	1.0
MCV (fL)	50–68	60	Neutrophil (mature)	28–47	37.0
MCH (pg)	17.0–21.0	19.0	Lymphocyte	39–62	53.0
MCHC (%)	30.0–34.0	32.0	Monocyte	2–10	5.0
Reticulocytes (%)	0.0–1.0	0.4	Eosinophil	0.5–11	3.5
ESR (mm in 1 hour)	Variable	—	Basophil	0–2	0.5
RBC diameter (μm)	4.0–8.0	6.0	—	—	—

Abbreviations: ESR, erythrocyte sedimentation rate; MCH, mean cell hemoglobin; MCHC, mean cell hemoglobin concentration; RBC, red blood cell.

Data from Thorn CE. Normal hematology of the pig. In: Feldman B, Zinkl J, Jain N, editors. Schalm's veterinary hematology. 5th edition. Philadelphia: Lippincott, Williams & Wilkins; 2000. p. 1089–95.

Leukocytes

The neutrophils of pigs, being 12 to 15 μm in diameter, have irregularly stained nuclei with irregular margins [8,10]. They have an irregular nuclear membrane and moderately coarse chromatin with well-defined lobes [10]. The cytoplasm of porcine neutrophils stains a pale pink to blue and contains small pink granules with Romanowsky stains [8,10,19]. Band neutrophils have a U-shaped nucleus and may be present in the healthy animal [10,11]. Metamyelocytes have a less mature chromatin pattern, and nuclear shape may vary from kidney bean shaped to a ring form with no lobation, with the cytoplasm staining a pale blue [10].

The nuclei of porcine eosinophils are poorly segmented and may appear immature [10]. They have round to oval organ cytoplasmic granules, and the nucleus often appears to be a band [8]. According to Thorn [10], the cytoplasmic granules are round to oval, stain a pale orange, and tend to fill the cytoplasm. The basophil nucleus stains lavender and has a smooth chromatin pattern. The cytoplasmic granules of the basophil are coccoid to dumbbell shaped and stain similar to or more intensely than the nucleus.

The neutrophil concentration is less than the lymphocyte concentration of healthy pigs [10]. Small lymphocytes are 7 to 10 μm in diameter. They have a round to oval nucleus with a condensed chromatin pattern and a small rim of pale blue cytoplasm [8]. Large lymphocytes are 11 to 15 μm in diameter with a chromatin pattern that is slightly coarse and does not stain as intensely as the small lymphocyte [8,10,19]. According to Campbell [8], large lymphocytes may contain low numbers of round to oblong azurophilic granules usually located at the margin of the cell.

Monocytes are similar in size to large lymphocytes with a diameter of 14 to 18 μm. They have a convoluted nucleus with lacy chromatin, often with localized condensation [8]. The cytoplasm may contain granules or vacuoles. Even with careful observation, some monocytes may be difficult to distinguish from a large lymphocyte or immature neutrophils [8–11].

Factors affecting the hemogram

There are numerous factors that can affect the interpretation of the hemogram, including age, gender, physiologic state, season, nutrition, and environmental condition [19]. Newborn piglets have a high PCV. During the first week of life, there is a 30% reduction in red blood cell numbers and a 38% decrease in red cell mass because of the increase in the amount of plasma volume from absorption of colostrum [20]. The blood volume of the young pig is the greatest it is ever going to be and decreases with age [19].

At birth, the percentage of neutrophils is approximately 60% to 85% of the white blood cells (WBCs) [19]. Lymphocytes are only approximately 20% of WBCs. Within 2 weeks of birth, neutrophil numbers begin to decrease and lymphocyte numbers increase and remain so for the rest of the animal's life [8,10]. This is similar to many other species that have a low neutrophil to lymphocyte (N/L) ratio, 0.7:1 [10]. This is important when examining hemograms of animals with inflammatory diseases. Minipigs mount a lower leukocyte response than animals with high N/L ratios and inflammatory diseases, and they may show only a reversal of the N/L ratio with mild inflammatory diseases. Marked neutrophilia is associated with more severe inflammatory diseases [8,22].

In general, the WBCs of swine behave similar to those of other species with respect to infectious processes [8,10,11,22]. Neutrophilia is observed when pigs have bacterial infections, typically with a left shift.

As in many species, endotoxemia induces a host of biochemical mediators in pigs leading to significant cardiovascular and hematologic changes. Infusion of endotoxin (ie, lipopolysaccharide) results in changes in the swine hemogram, such as granulocytopenia and thrombocytopenia [23,24]. Typically, endotoxemia causes hemoconcentration, leukocytopenia, and thrombocytopenia in swine [25].

With viral diseases, the WBCs counts of swine decline, accounted for by a granulocytopenia [19,26,27], and an increase of immature neutrophils in peripheral blood can be seen with severe infections [19].

Various forms of neoplasia are commonly observed in geriatric potbellied pigs. Lymphoma and lymphosarcomas would increase the WBC count by increasing the number of lymphoblasts and poorly differentiated lymphocytes in the circulation [8].

Disorders that cause anemia in swine

Although not a comprehensive list, Table 2 outlines several causes of anemia in swine and respective clinical signs, criteria for diagnosis, and recommended treatment.

Mineral and vitamin deficiencies

The primary cause of anemia in suckling piglets is iron-deficiency anemia, because milk is low in iron. These neonates have hemoglobin levels ranging from 10 to 12 g/dL of blood, and their average total body iron content is approximately 50 mg [9]. Piglets require iron at a rate of 1 mg/day and can develop anemia within 10 to 14 days after birth without supplementation [28]. Because the piglets grow rapidly, they deplete the available iron, which is only approximately 10% of the total body iron content and become anemic during the first 1 to 2 weeks. Iron deficiency in swine results in a microcytic hypochromic anemia as in other species, characterized by reduced hemoglobin, hematocrit, and red blood cell count. Clumping of erythroblastic cells in the bone marrow has been associated with iron deficiency [29]. Reduced serum iron and percent transferrin saturation may also occur. A deficiency of iron may also affect the immune system. It has been demonstrated that unsupplemented piglets have decreased neutrophils and circulating B lymphocytes [28]. Domestic pigs are supplemented with iron by means of intramuscular injection on days 1 to 3 after birth. This procedure can be adapted to potbellied pigs if they do not have access to soil early in life. Soil can be a good source of iron that piglets can ingest by rooting around early in life.

Copper promotes iron absorption and heme production. Consequently, copper deficiency results in an iron-deficiency anemia. Excesses of copper and cobalt can also result in anemia [29]. An excess of iodine can result in reduced liver iron and reduced hemoglobin [29]. A high intake of selenium for longer than 30 days can result in anemia in swine [30].

Deficiencies of niacin (vitamin B_3), pantothenic acid (vitamin B_5), pyridoxine (vitamin B_6), folic acid (vitamin B_9), and cobalamin (vitamin B_{12}) can all result in normocytic anemia. A lack of sufficient vitamin C can reduce use of folic acid and vitamin B_{12}, leading to anemia that can be compounded by reduced iron absorption [31]. A zinc deficiency may also result in reduced hemoglobin and red blood cell count.

Most mineral and vitamin deficiencies can be prevented in the potbellied pig by feeding age-appropriate commercially prepared diets. Healthy pet pig diets may include supplementation of fruits, vegetables, and pasture grazing. Heavy dietary proportions of table scraps and other companion animal treats may lead to vitamin and mineral imbalances.

Toxicities

Mycotoxin toxicities can cause changes in the hemogram, such as hemoconcentration from dehydration or anemia from blood loss. Aflatoxicosis can cause a decrease in liver production of clotting factors, resulting in hemorrhaging. Affected swine may have hemorrhages in the pleural and peritoneal cavities [32].

Anticoagulant rodenticide toxicity can occur after a single dose of warfarin at 3 mg/kg of body weight. Chronic exposures of small dosages (ie, 0.05 mg/kg/d over 7 days) can also produce toxicosis. Mild to severe hemorrhaging may lead to blood loss anemia with increases in prothrombin time and activated partial prothrombin clotting times Treatment includes supplementation with injectable and oral vitamin K [33].

Infectious diseases

Mycoplasma suis (*Eperythrozoon suis*) is a blood-borne bacterium that causes anemia in swine breeds. The bacteria attach to red blood cell walls, resulting in damage to erythrocytes and subsequent hemolytic anemia. This disease, also known as porcine eperythrozoonosis (PE), is characterized by acute normochromic normocytic anemia, fever, and icterus [34,35]. In piglets, the disease is also characterized by depression, muscle weakness, and poor weight gain.

Table 2
Disorders that cause anemia in swine

Disorder	Ages affected	Other clinical signs	Diagnosis	Treatment	Prognosis
Gastric ulcer	Older growing pigs and adults	Inappetence, weight loss, bruxism; normal feces or firm, dark, and tarry	History and clinical signs. Endoscopy	Cimetidine or ranitidine, omeprazole, bismuth salicylate	Varies from poor to fair; depends on severity
Iron deficiency	Nursery pigs	Slower growth rate and rough hair coat	Hematology, history, and absence of other lesions	200-mg iron injection on days 1 through 3 of age	Good
Sarcoptes scabiei	Nursery pigs to adults	Scratching and rubbing against walls, rough hair coat, keratinization of skin	Deep skin scraping from the ear canal	Ivermectin	Good; depends on the severity (may need >1 treatment)
Trichuris suis	2–6 months old	Anorexia, diarrhea with mucus, dark feces or melena	Response to treatment	Ivermectin	Good
Hemorrhagic ileitis	4–6 months old	Bleeding from the anus, usually with normal body condition	Clinical signs	Tylosin	Fair to good; this depends on degree of anemia
Proliferative enteritis	2–5 months old	Various degrees of weight loss and anorexia, black tarry feces to frank blood	Endoscopy, biopsy	Tylosin, Carbadex	Fair to good; this depends on degree of anemia

					Fair to good; this depends on degree of anemia
Porcine eperythrozoonosis	2 months up to adults	Lethargy, reduced growth, occasional icterus	Stained blood smear to demonstrate organism, indirect HA titer of 1:80 or higher	Tetracycline, chlortetracycline	Fair to good; this depends on degree of anemia
Aflatoxin	All ages	Depression, anorexia, ascites, elevated liver enzymes, occasional icterus	Liver enzymes elevated with clinical signs, feed analysis for toxin	Change feed	Fair; this depends on the length on the feed
Tricothecenes	All ages	Gastroenteritis	Feed analysis for toxin	Change feed	Fair; this depends on the length on the feed
Zearalenone	All ages	Swollen vulvas and mammary glands in prepubertal gilts	Feed analysis for toxin	Change feed	Fair; this depends on the length on the feed
Warfarin toxicity	Any age	Lameness, stiff gait, lethargy, dark tarry feces	Prolonged clotting time, demonstrate toxin in blood and liver	Vitamin K	Fair; this depends on degree of anemia

Abbreviation: HA, hemagglutination.

Data from Straw BE, Dewey CE, Wilson MR. Differential diagnosis of swine diseases. In: Straw BE, editor. Diseases of swine. 8th edition. Ames (IA): Iowa State University Press; 1999. p. 41–86.

Porcine proliferative enteropathy caused by *Lawsonia intracellularis* can result in gastrointestinal bleeding because of extensive mucosal damage, leading to blood-loss anemia. These signs may also occur with hemorrhagic ileitis.

Parasitism

The ova of *Ascaris suum* can be ingested and result in infections that lead to anemia and eosinophilia in swine [19,36]. After ingestion of infective eggs, larvae hatch and migrate through the intestinal wall into the hepatic portal system. Migration through liver parenchyma causes hemorrhagic foci and systemic eosinophilia [37]. Larvae of the swine whipworm, *Trichuris suis*, penetrate and ulcerate intestinal mucosal lining with subsequent erosion of capillary beds, leading to hemorrhage and anemia [37].

Blood transfusion

In cases of severe blood loss, it may be necessary to restore circulating red blood cells and plasma volume by means of blood transfusion. A blood transfusion may be indicated in swine with acute hemorrhage from gastric or esophageal ulcers, umbilical hemorrhage in neonates, or gastrointestinal blood loss caused by proliferative enteropathy [38] or other conditions that result in severe anemia. Hemolytic reactions to transfusions rarely occur in pigs that have not been previously transfused. This may be attributable to low density of antigens on pig erythrocytes. It has been reported that disseminated intravascular coagulation (DIC) has resulted from swine that received A- through O-incompatible transfusions, however, purportedly as a result of recipient plasma anti-A antibodies reacting with A substance in the donor plasma [39]. In light of the potential severe plasma antibody interactions, Smith and colleagues [39] suggest transfusing packed red blood cells with a minimal volume of plasma or using cross-matched blood. This becomes particularly important if a pig may need repeated transfusions.

Swine have 16 recognized blood groups, A through O, with two or more alleles in each group [21,39]. In testing for blood compatibility, a serum agglutination test may not be sufficient, because many antibodies responsible for hemolytic transfusion reactions do not cause erythrocyte agglutination. Smith and colleagues [39] recommend that compatibility testing should include a standard saline agglutination method and an anti-pig immunoglobulin G (IgG) reagent–enhanced agglutination method.

The clinical parameters used in the decision to perform a blood transfusion have been described elsewhere for other species and may be used similarly in the pig. The amount of blood to transfuse to the swine patient can also be determined in a manner comparable to that in other species. When calculating blood deficit and volume of blood needed for deficit correction, consider that the normal blood volume in swine species is estimated to be 8% to 10% of body weight.

Administration of blood through an in-line filter and indwelling intravenous catheter is strongly recommended. When venous access cannot be gained, however, it is possible to administer blood by means of intraperitoneal injection. This method results in complete but delayed absorption of unaltered erythrocytes. Because this method does not provide immediate cardiovascular support, it is not recommended in cases of hypovolemic shock. Neither is intraperitoneal blood transfusion recommended in swine patients that have peritonitis, ascites, abdominal distention, or abdominal compromise of any kind [38].

References

[1] Boldrick L. Veterinary care of potbellied pigs. Orange (CA): All Publishing Company; 1993.

[2] Bradford JR. Caring for potbellied pigs. Vet Med 1991;86:1173–81.

[3] Braun WF, Casteel SW. Potbellied pigs: miniature porcine pets. Vet Clin North Am Small Anim Pract 1993;23:1149–77.

[4] Johnson L. Physical and chemical restraint of miniature pet pigs. In: Reeves DE, editor. Care and management of miniature pet pigs. Santa Barbara (CA): Veterinary Practice Publishing Company; 1993. p. 59–66.

[5] Tynes VV. Emergency care for potbellied pigs. Vet Clin North Am Exot Anim Pract 1998;1: 179–80.

[6] Tynes VV. Preventative health care for pet potbellied pigs. Vet Clin North Am Exot Anim Pract 1999;2:495–510.

[7] Lawhorn B. Diseases and conditions of miniature pet pigs. In: Reeves DE, editor. Care and management of miniature pet pigs. Santa Barbara (CA): Veterinary Practice Publishing Company; 1993. p. 77–101.

[8] Campbell TW. Mammalian hematology: laboratory animals and miscellaneous species. In: Thrall MA, editor. Veterinary hematology and clinical chemistry. Ames (IA): Blackwell Publishing; 2006. p. 211–24.

[9] Jain NC. Essentials of veterinary hematology. Philadephia: Lea & Febiger; 1993.

[10] Thorn CE. Normal hematology of the pig. In: Feldman B, Zinkl J, Jain N, editors. Schalm's veterinary hematology. 5th edition. Philadelphia: Lippincott, Williams and Wilkins; 2000. p. 1089–95.

[11] Thrall MA, Weiser G, Jain N. Laboratory evaluation of bone marrow. In: Thrall MA, editor. Veterinary hematology and clinical chemistry. Ames (IA): Blackwell Publishing; 2006. p. 149–78.

[12] Hu C, Cheang A, Retnam L, et al. A simple technique for blood collection in the pig. Lab Anim 1993;27:364–7.

[13] Lawhorn B. A new approach for obtaining blood samples from pigs. J Am Vet Med Assoc 1988;192:781–2.

[14] Muirhead MR. Blood sampling in pigs. In Pract 1981;3:16–32.

[15] Westercamp D. Venipuncture in miniature pet pigs. In: Reeves DE, editor. Care and management of miniature pet pigs. Santa Barbara (CA): Veterinary Practice Publishing Company; 1993. p. 51–8.

[16] Spellman P. Sedation of pot-bellied pigs. Vet Rec 1999;145:56.

[17] Snook CS. Use of subcutaneous abdominal vein for blood sampling and intravenous catheterization in potbellied pigs. J Am Vet Med Assoc 2001;219:809–10.

[18] Straw BE, Meuten DJ, Thacker BJ. Physical examination. In: Straw BE, editor. Diseases of swine. 8th edition. Ames (IA): Iowa State University Press; 1999. p. 15–7.

[19] Huhn RG, Osweiler GD, Switzer WP. Application of the orbital sinus bleeding technique to swine. Lab Anim Care 1969;19:403–5.

[20] Evans EW. Interpretation of porcine leukocyte responses. In: Feldman B, Zinkl J, Jain N, editors. Schalm's veterinary hematology. 5th edition. Philadelphia: Lippincott, Williams and Wilkins; 2000. p. 411–6.

[21] Cooper KC. Porcine red blood cells as a source of blood transfusions in humans. Xenotransplantation 2003;10:383–6.

[22] Egeli AK, Framstad T, Morberg H. Clinical biochemistry, haematology and body weight in piglets. Acta Vet Scand 1998;39:381–93.

[23] Lofstedt J, Roth JA, Ross RF, et al. Depression of polymorphonuclear leukocyte function associated with experimentally induced Escherichia coli mastitis in sows. Am J Vet Res 1983; 44:1224–8.

[24] Olson NC. Porcine endotoxemia: chemical mediators and therapeutic interventions. In: Tumbleson ME, Schook LB, editors. Advances in swine in biomedical research, vol. 1. New York: Plenum Press; 1996. p. 19–32.

[25] Naess F, Roeise O, Pillgram-Larsen J, et al. Plasma proteolysis and circulating cells in relation to varying endotoxin concentrations in porcine endotoxemia. Circ Shock 1989;28(2): 89–100.

[26] Page GR, Wang F, Hahn EC. Interaction of pseudorabies virus with porcine peripheral blood lymphocytes. J Leukoc Biol 1992;52:441–8.

[27] Knudsen RC, Genovesi EV. In vivo and vitro effects of moderately virulent African swine fever virus on mitogenesis of pig lymphocytes. Vet Immunol Immunopathol 1987;15(4): 323–36.

[28] Svoboda M, Drabek J, Krejci J, et al. Impairment of the peripheral lymphoid compartment in iron-deficient piglets. J Vet Med B Infect Dis Vet Public Health 2004;51:231–7.

[29] Reese DE. Nutrient deficiencies and excesses. In: Straw BE, editor. Diseases of swine. 8th edition. Ames (IA): Iowa State University Press; 1999. p. 743–55.

[30] Hall JO. Selenium. In: Gupta RC, editor. Veterinary toxicology: basic and clinical principles. New York: Academic Press; 2007. p. 453–60.

[31] Blair R, Newsome F. Involvement of water-soluble vitamins in diseases of swine. J Anim Sci 1985;60(6):1508–17.

[32] Coppock RW, Christian RG. Aflatoxins. In: Gupta RC, editor. Veterinary toxicology: basic and clinical principles. New York: Academic Press; 2007. p. 939–50.

[33] Carson TL. Toxic minerals, chemicals, plants, and gases. In: Straw BE, D'Allaire D, Mengellins WL, et al, editors. Diseases of swine. 8th edition. Ames (IA): Iowa State University Press; 1999. p. 783–96.

[34] Heinritzi K. Eperythrozoonosis. In: Straw BE, D'Allaire D, Mengellins WL, et al, editors. Diseases of swine. 8th edition. Ames (IA): Iowa State University Press; 1999. p. 413–8.

[35] Hoelzle LE, Adelt D, Hoelzle K, et al. Development of a diagnostic PCR assay based on novel DNA sequences for the detection of Mycoplasma suis (Eperythrozoon suis) in porcine blood. Vet Microbiol 2003;93:185–96.

[36] Reeves DE. Parasite control in miniature pet pigs. In: Reeves DE, editor. Care and management of miniature pet pigs. Santa Barbara (CA): Veterinary Practice Publishing Company; 1993. p. 101–7.

[37] Corwin RM, Stewart TB. Internal parasites. In: Straw BE, D'Allaire D, Mengellins WL, et al, editors. Diseases of swine. 8th edition. Ames (IA): Iowa State University Press; 1999. p. 713–30.

[38] Radostits RM, Gay CC, Blood DC, et al, editors. Veterinary medicine: a textbook of the diseases of cattle, sheep, pigs, goats, and horses. 9th edition. New York: WB Saunders; 2000. p. 404–6.

[39] Smith DM, Newhouse M, Naziruddin B, et al. Blood groups and transfusions in pigs. Xenotransplantation 2006;13:186–94.

VETERINARY
CLINICS
Exotic Animal Practice

ELSEVIER
SAUNDERS

Vet Clin Exot Anim 11 (2008) 583–595

Flow Cytometry Applications for Exotic Animals

Stephen A. Kania, MS, PhD

*Department of Comparative Medicine, College of Veterinary Medicine, University
of Tennessee, 2407 River Drive, Knoxville, TN 37849, USA*

Flow cytometry has become an important tool in hematology for the characterization of cell populations. It is used to study immunologic relations of different animal species, mechanisms of immunity, and disease mechanisms. It is useful for diagnosis of disease in individuals, for comparative and evolutionary studies, and to examine the effects of environmental factors and toxins. Specific applications of flow cytometry in hematology include but are not limited to diagnosis of lymphoid malignancy, acquired and inherited immune deficiency, immune dysfunction, lymphocyte function, neutrophil function, immune-mediated hemolytic anemia, and immune-mediated thrombocytopenia.

Flow cytometers analyze individual cells, and because this process is rapid, it is possible to collect information from large numbers of cells within individual samples. Flow cytometry complements and has advantages over other methods of cell analysis, such as immunohistochemistry and cytologic examination of cells stained with Wright stain (or modifications of Wright stain) and examined microscopically. This includes the ability to determine multiple parameters of individual cells, objective analysis, and speed. Flow cytometry is a standard diagnostic resource in human medicine [1], has taken on an important role in veterinary medicine [2], and is increasingly applied for diagnostic and research applications for exotic animals and wildlife.

Methods and mechanisms

An overview of how flow cytometers function should serve to explain their capabilities and limitations for hematology applications. The

E-mail address: skania@utk.edu

1094-9194/08/$ - see front matter © 2008 Elsevier Inc. All rights reserved.
doi:10.1016/j.cvex.2008.03.002   *vetexotic.theclinics.com*

instruments come in a variety of models that differ in the way they transport cells (fluidics), their laser light sources, signal processing, and software systems. Most flow cytometers share some common basic functions. They have a system for streaming individual cells into a chamber (flow cell) through which a focused laser light shines. As occurs when a flashlight shines on a ball in the dark, a shadow is produced proportionate to the size of the cell in the chamber (forward scatter) and light is deflected to the sides of the cell, providing information about its structure. Just as the surface of a tennis ball would have a different pattern of light deflected to the side than a smooth-surfaced orange, a granulocyte deflects more light than an erythrocyte, and thus has more side scatter. These two features, forward scatter and side scatter, are used to "divide" populations of cells into sets, such as erythrocytes, lymphocytes, monocytes, and granulocytes (Fig. 1). In analytic instruments, this division is an information processing event and is used for the analysis of data rather than as a physical separation of cells. Cell sorters, used primarily for research, can use these parameters to separate cells physically. Probes, often antibodies tagged with fluorescent markers, are used to identify and divide populations of cells further (Fig. 2). Laser light energizes the fluorescent tag, stimulating it to emit light. A system of filters separates the light, based on its wavelength(s), and distributes it to sensors that amplify the signal and transmit this information to a central processing unit. The amount of emitted light coming from each cell is measured. Cells emitting significantly more light than control cells are considered positive. This information is used to enumerate populations and subpopulations of cells, for example, to determine the number of CD4 antigen-positive (CD4+) helper T-cell lymphocytes in a population of leukocytes based on the binding of fluorescein-tagged anti-CD4 antibody bound to the cells. Computer analysis adds an important capability to flow cytometry. The forward scatter and side scatter information used to identify lymphocytes can be combined with antibody binding information

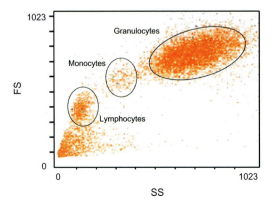

Fig. 1. Plot of blood forward scatter (FS) and side scatter (SS).

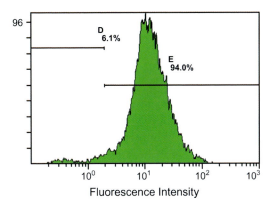

Fig. 2. Surface-bound immunoglobulin G. (D, baseline fluorescence; E, IgG surface positive cells).

to, for example, determine not only the number of CD4+ cells in blood but the proportion of CD4+ cells within the population of lymphocytes. The process of cell analysis occurs at the rate of hundreds of cells analyzed per second. As such, it is practical to analyze large numbers of cells, typically 10,000 to 20,000, for each sample. Most flow cytometers can distinguish fluorescent light emitted at more than one wavelength. Using this capability, helper T cells can be identified with a fluorescein-tagged antibody that binds to CD4 lymphocytes and, in the same sample, cytotoxic T cells can be labeled with a phycoerythrin-tagged antibody that recognizes CD8+ lymphocytes. Thus, the percentage of CD4+ and CD8+ cells can be determined within a single tube of cells. Depending on the instrument's capabilities, it may be able to analyze information from four or more fluorescent tags. Using multiparametric analysis, helper T cells can be distinguished from B cells and the concentration of major histocompatibility complex (MHC) II antigen on the surface of each population of cells can be measured.

Standardized cell processing procedures and gating techniques have been recommended for use in veterinary medicine [3,4]. There are no universally accepted procedures, however, and different instruments, software, cell processing procedures, methods for establishing gates, and reagents hamper comparisons of data among laboratories.

The example presented in this section describes the most common clinical use of flow cytometry, the enumeration of leukocyte populations and sub-populations. Flow cytometry has a wide range of applications, which are described further. This serves, however, to highlight the key features of flow cytometry. Cells are interrogated, individually, with a finely focused beam of laser light; their relative size and granularity are determined; fluorescence intensity information can be obtained for binding of one or more probes; and software is used to combine selected characteristics for sample analysis.

Antibodies for exotic animal studies

Immunophenotyping leukocytes and other common flow cytometry applications require antibodies that bind specifically to cell surface markers. Conventions are used for naming cell surface components, and one commonly used for flow cytometry is the assignment of cluster of differentiation (CD) antigen numbers [5]. A single CD designation is used for all antibodies that react with the same cell antigen. Human leukocyte antigens have been assigned through at least CD339 but with some skipped numbers and some subdivided. Corresponding antigens may not exist or be identified for nonhuman species. When known, the markers are correlated with specific cellular functions. Antibodies reactive with a coreceptor for MHC class I molecules identify CD8+ cytotoxic T cells. Anti-CD79 binds to lymphocytes with B-cell antigen receptors. Other antibodies recognize families of cells. Anti-CD3 is broadly reactive with T cells, and anti-CD5 reacts with T cells and a subset of B cells. Antibodies are available for the most clinically important human leukocyte markers, and many markers are available for mice, companion animals, and other commercially important animals. These are primarily monoclonal antibodies produced from hybridomas generated from mice or other rodents. Thus, the antibodies originate from a single splenocyte. They are highly specific, reacting with a single epitope. As such, a given monoclonal antibody may react with target cells from a single species of animal. Its epitope, however, may be conserved on cells of related species and may be present on cells of diverse species. For example, monoclonal antibody CA2.1D6 produced against canine immunogen (P.F. Moore, University of California at Davis, personal communication, 2007) reacts with canine and feline B cells.

Antibodies used for exotic animals are produced against the species of interest or, more often, are cross-reactive with other animal species. Production of specific antibodies requires screening, identification, and characterization procedures that are labor-intensive and expensive. To characterize the binding of monoclonal anti-CD45R to cetacean lymphocytes, De Guise and colleagues [6] immunoprecipitated labeled antigen, identified its reactivity on lymph node and thymus sections with immunohistochemistry, and examined its expression on cells from various tissues using flow cytometry.

Comprehensive wildlife studies often require using a panel of antibodies that may include antibodies prepared against more than one species of animal. In a study of beluga whale (*Delphinapterus leucas*) lymphocytes, Bernier and colleagues [7] used anti-mouse immunoglobulin (Ig) M, anti-human CD4, and anti-bovine MHC II. Likewise, to study sea otter lymphocytes, Schwartz and colleagues [8] used rat anti-mouse CD3, mouse anti-human CD79, and mouse anti-bovine MHC II.

The easiest way to obtain antibodies for studies of wildlife species for which antibodies have not been produced is to use cross-reactive antibodies previously identified for that species or a closely related species. Several studies have been undertaken to identify cross-reactive antibodies. Some are limited to domestic animals, whereas others examine cross-reactivities with exotic species. This information can be accessed in databases, workshop reports, and journal publications. An extensive searchable list of antibodies and their suppliers is available from the free on-line "Linscott's Directory of Immunological and Biological Reagents." This resource includes cross-reactivity information when provided by suppliers. Veterinary Medical Research and Diagnostics (VMRD; Pullman, Washington) provides cross-reactivity information with animals, including cattle, goat, sheep, swine, horse, cat, dog, ferret, mink, human being, mouse, and rabbit. The Washington State University Monoclonal Antibody Center in the College of Veterinary Medicine maintains a Web site listing antibodies reactive with selected mammals, fish, birds, amphibians, and other species. The US Veterinary Immune Reagent Network [9] is developing reagents reactive with the major leukocyte subpopulations of catfish, equine, poultry, ruminants, swine, and trout. The animal homolog section of the Human Leukocyte Differentiation Antigen 8 Workshop reported the results of cross-reactivity testing of 376 monoclonal antibodies with 16 species, including nonhuman primates, ruminants, swine, horse, carnivores, rabbit, guinea pig, chicken, and fish [10]. Whatever the source, care should be taken to use antibodies of known specificity, proved to be useful for flow cytometry. Antibodies for other applications, such as immunohistochemistry, may not react with native cell surface antigens.

Antibodies against immunoglobulins are often more readily available and easier to characterize than antibodies produced against CD antigens. They are used to detect surface immunoglobulins, which serve as receptors on B cells and are immunoglobulin bound to cells in autoimmune conditions. Monoclonal antibodies have been developed to trout (*Salmo gairdneri*) IgM and used for flow cytometry to characterize the size of trout B cells [11]. Milston and colleagues [12] validated the reactivity of anti-trout IgM with Chinook salmon (*Oncorhynchus tshawytscha*) IgM and used it to enumerate salmon (*Oncorhynchus tshawytscha*) B cells. Ronneseth and colleagues [13] used rabbit anti-cod IgM to identify cod B cells and monoclonal antibody to identify neutrophils. They determined the proportions of these leukocytes in head, kidney, blood, and spleen and found a high proportion of neutrophils in peripheral blood. This approach was used, with affinity-purified rabbit anti-dolphin immunoglobulin, to determine that bottlenose dolphins (*Tursiops truncates*) have ratios of B cells to T cells in blood similar to those of other mammals [14].

Immune-mediated thrombocytopenia, resulting from autoimmune antibodies binding to platelets, and immune-mediated hemolytic anemia, resulting from antibodies bound to erythrocytes, are diagnosed by detection of deposited antibody and complement (Fig. 3). Flow cytometry may provide the most sensitive method of detection for these conditions [15,16]. This

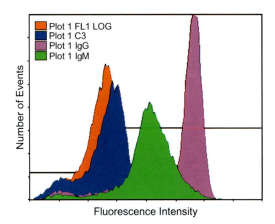

Fig. 3. Erythrocytes positive for IgG and IgM and negative for the third component of complement.

methodology has been used for companion animals but is not yet in widespread use for exotics.

Immunophenotyping

The enumeration of cell populations identified with antibodies is probably the most frequently used hematologic application of flow cytometry. Immunophenotying is used to identify and count cell populations and subpopulations. The information obtained from this analysis can be key to the diagnosis of primary or acquired immune deficiencies, immune dysfunction, and detection and characterization of malignancies. It is commonly used for the identification of abnormal populations of cells in blood in cases of leukocytosis and in tissue masses, especially when lymphoid neoplasia is suspected. Lymphomas have been identified in human beings, companion animals, and exotic animals, including badgers (*Meles meles*), mink (*Mustela vison*), striped skunk (*Mephitis mephitis*), ferrets (*Mustela putorius furo*), sea otters (*Enhydra lutris*) [17], and camels (*Camelus dromedaries*) [18]. Complete blood cell counts with differentials from blood smears or hematology instruments provide information about numbers of cell types, such as lymphocytes, monocytes, and neutrophils. As mentioned previously, flow cytometry uses physical characteristics and cell type–specific antibodies to identify subpopulations of cells. The targets of detecting antibodies include CD antigens and other functional molecules. Thus, lymphocytes can be further subdivided into CD4+ (helper T cells), CD8+ (cytotoxic T cells), and CD21+ (B cells). Lymphoid neoplasias often result from the malignant transformation of a single cell. Their clonal progeny have the same antigenic characteristics, and thus the same surface marker profile. Consequently, a fine needle aspirate from an enlarged lymph node that contains 90%

CD4+ cells and few CD8+ or B cells shows an abnormally high proportion of one cell subtype, suggesting the possibility of clonal expansion of CD4+ cells compatible with a lymphosarcoma.

Malignant cells sometimes exhibit antigenic infidelity with aberrant expression of cell surface markers [1]. For example, B cells may produce T-cell antigens or vice versa, resulting in coexpression of T-cell and B-cell markers as has also been observed with canine lymphomas and leukemias [19]. As with all laboratory findings, flow cytometry results from leukocytosis must be interpreted in the context of the patient's history and other test results. DNA-based clonality testing using the polymerase chain reaction, available for some species of animals, may provide additional useful information [20].

Immunodeficiency

Flow cytometry is useful for the diagnosis of most acquired and primary immunodeficiencies. It has played a key role in determining the effects of lentiviruses in the family Retroviridae on the immune systems of their hosts. Feline immunodeficiency virus (FIV)–infected domestic cats show a gradual decrease in their number of CD4+ cells compared with CD8+ lymphocytes [21–23]. This generally occurs because of a decrease in CD4+ cells. The long-term effects of FIV or related lentiviruses on the health of nondomestic felids have not been elucidated. Flow cytometry studies of infected animals seem to shed some light on the pathomechanism of infection in these animals. Captive lions (*Panthera leo*) infected with immunodeficiency virus as determined with commercial serologic testing and Western blot analysis, show a decrease in CD4+ cells [24]. It is accompanied, however, by a decrease in CD8+ lymphocytes. Thus, it seems that a general loss of lymphocytes occurs during immunodeficiency virus infection in lions. Wild lions and pumas (*Puma concolor*) serologically positive for immunodeficiency virus exposure also show a decrease in CD4+ cells, along with a decline in CD8+ lymphocytes strongly reactive with anti-CD8β [25]. These studies, performed with monoclonal antibodies developed against domestic cat lymphocytes, suggest that FIV and similar viruses infecting exotic felids have a long-term effect on lymphocyte subsets not seen in uninfected felids and demonstrate the value of flow cytometry on hematologic studies of wildlife. Immunodeficiency viruses do not universally produce a sustained decrease in CD4+ cells. Bovine immunodeficiency virus seems to have a significant but mild and transient effect on CD4/CD8 subset ratios in cattle [26].

Flow cytometry is also used for diagnosis of primary immunodeficiencies. Several immunodeficiencies have been described in human beings, resulting in abnormal numbers of lymphocytes or lymphocyte subsets. These include class I and II bare lymphocyte syndromes, severe combined immunodeficiency (SCID), and X-linked immunoproliferative syndrome. These disorders are characterized by few or no circulating CD8+ lymphocytes,

CD4+ lymphocytes, T and B lymphocytes, and unregulated B-cell growth, respectively. The mechanisms and range of effects of these syndromes affecting people have recently been reviewed [27]. Fewer primary immune deficiencies have been reported in veterinary medicine. They may be attributed to failure-to-thrive syndromes without an underlying cause being determined. Canine X-linked severe combined immunodeficiency (XSCID) is characterized by stunted growth and susceptibility to life-threatening infection [28]. Neonates that have XSCID have low but nearly normal lymphocyte counts, however. Flow cytometry can be used to characterize the elevated B cells and scant or absent T cells present in the blood of these dogs. Some dogs, however, may have nearly normal numbers of T cells [29]. Autosomal recessive SCID of Jack Russell terriers presents with a lack of B cells and T cells [30], and equine and mouse SCID has the same presentation [31]. There are few if any reports of primary immune deficiency in exotic animals, probably because of a lack of surveillance and short survival time.

Use of dyes to identify cell populations

For exotic animals, identification of cells with dyes offers a potential alternative for the enumeration of cell populations when antibodies are not available for the species being studied. A fluorescent lipophilic dye, 3,3'-dihexlyoxacarbocyanine iodide ($DiOC_6$), binds to cells and produces different fluorescence patterns with different types of cells. It has been shown to be useful for blood from quail (*Coturnix coturnix japonica*) [32] and for bone marrow from rats, mice, dogs, and monkeys [33]. In fish blood, absolute numbers of erythrocytes, granulocytes, monocytes, and lymphocytes were enumerated with this technique. In the same study, $DiOC_6$ was applied successfully to goldfish, loach, eel, rainbow trout, and iguana [34]. This dye is readily available, and the staining procedure is quick and easy to perform. The greatest obstacle in applying this technique to new species is the process of correlating populations of cells identified by their fluorescence intensity and scatter characteristics with particular cell types.

Cell surface expression of major histocompatibility complex molecules

In addition to enumerating cell populations, flow cytometry is used to determine levels of protein expression, especially of cell surface molecules. Stimulation of antigen-presenting cells leads to increased expression of MHC molecules on the cell surface. Class II MHC proteins present exogenously produced antigens to T-helper cells stimulating downstream events, including T-cell help to B cells and generation of a cytotoxic T-cell response. Use of flow cytometry to measure class II MHC production can be an important indicator of response to vaccination, as shown in reindeer (*Rangifer tarandus*) [35]. Expression of MHC class II on the surface of T cells from beluga whales (*Delphinapterus leucas*) is upregulated by mitogenic stimulation, resulting in increased density [7].

Phagocyte function

Phagocyte function is a useful indicator of the status of important components of the innate immune system. Since Metchnikoff's discovery of phagocytosis in invertebrates, it has been found to play an important role in the protection of a wide range of animals. For analysis of immune function, two activities, phagocytosis and oxidative burst, can be measured separately. The ability of neutrophils, monocytes, or equivalent phagocytic cells to generate an oxidative burst in response to stimulation with a soluble agent, phorbol 12-myristate 13-acetate (PMA), is measured in addition to a particulate stimulant (*Escherichi coli*). Phagocytosis of opsonized fluorescein-conjugated *E coli* or beads is used. Both tests of phagocytic function can be performed using flow cytometry with commercial kits (Orpegen Pharma, Heidelberg, Germany) or with noncommercial reagents. They provide information about the percentage of host cells capable of phagocytizing and the number of phagocytized particles, the number of phagocytic cells generating an oxidative burst, and the strength of the burst response. These tests do not require species-specific reagents and have been successfully applied to a wide range of animals. Phagocytosis and oxidative burst tests were used with Tiger salamanders (*Ambystoma tigrinum*) [28]. Treatment of the salamanders with dexamethasone reduced phagocytic activity. Thus, this may serve as an important measure of the effect of environmental factors on the immune system of vertebrate animals [36,37]. Incubations with mammalian cells are usually performed at 37°C, although it may be possible to use room temperature incubations for field experiments when temperature control is not possible [38]. Poikilotherms, such as fish [39], and other nonmammalian species may require lower temperatures and longer incubation times for optimal phagocytosis. Phagocytosis studies in birds can be performed using room temperature incubations [40]; however, it is the author's experience that the optimal temperature for psittacine phagocytosis is 41°C. De Guise and colleagues [41] used flow with 1-µM diameter fluorescent latex beads to measure phagocytosis in killer whale neutrophils. This technique was found to be convenient for studies of loons and other birds [40]. It did fail, however, to show significant effects of methylmercury exposure on birds, even though responses were suppressed when isolated leukocytes were used.

Lymphocyte blastogenesis

Measurement of lymphocyte responses to mitogenic and antigenic stimulation is an important index of immune function. It is used to determine primary or acquired immunodeficiencies in patients and responses of populations to environmental factors. This assay can be performed in a variety of different ways. The incorporation of tritiated thymidine into cell DNA is a standard for the measurement of blastogenesis. This method was directly compared with interleukin-2 receptor expression in the harbor seal (*Phoca vitulina*) using flow cytometric detection of phycoerythrin-conjugated human recombinant interleukin-2 [42]. The assays had good overall agreement, and differences between the assays were attributed to the measurement of somewhat different parameters.

The use of flow cytometry to measure lymphocyte responses to mitogenic stimulation has the advantages of not requiring radioactive materials and scintillation fluids or radiation detectors. The two tests provide equivalent results for at least some applications, and in addition to overall proliferative responses, subpopulations of lymphocytes can be examined [43]. Lymphocytes are separated using lymphocyte separation medium and then labeled with 5,6-carboxyfluorescein diacetate succinimidyl ester (CFSE) [44] and incubated with mitogenic stimulants. As the cells divide, each daughter cell receives half of the label. Thus, cell proliferation is measured as a decrease in dye content within each daughter cell. This test has been used with a variety of species, including snapper (*Pagrus auratus*) [45]. In this study, snapper peripheral blood lymphocytes were stimulated with lipopolysaccharide (LPS), phytohemagglutinin (PHA), and LPS combined with PHA. This proliferation assay was combined with surface marker identification to determine the proliferating populations of cells.

When lymphocytes are stimulated to undergo blastogenesis, their forward scatter and side scatter values increase. These changes have been used to measure the response of Chinook salmon (*Oncorhynchus tshawytscha*) B cells to stimulation with LPS [12].

Sample collection and submission

Instructions for sample collection, storage, and shipping of blood and other samples for flow cytometry testing should be obtained from the flow cytometry clinical laboratory to which samples are submitted. The availability of reagents to test wildlife and exotic animals and standard ranges should also be determined by contacting the laboratory. The condition of samples when they arrive for analysis has an impact on the usefulness of the information obtained. Flow cytometers require single-cell suspensions, and blood and aspirates are commonly tested. Products are available that extend the usefulness of blood collected for immunophenotyping (Cyto-Chex; Streck, Omaha, Nebraska). For field collections, when samples must be stored frozen, cryopreservatives have been found to preserve antigenic properties. The utility of cell preservatives should be determined for each marker being examined [46]. Fine needle aspirates should be obtained with minimal blood contamination. Cells from aspirates for immunophenotyping may be stored in buffered saline. Blood collected for phagocyte function assays is usually collected in heparin and needs to remain viable. All samples should be transported as rapidly as possible for processing and analysis. Extreme temperatures should be avoided, and samples should never be frozen without a cryopreservative.

Summary

Flow cytometry complements and extends the capabilities of traditional methods of hematologic testing. It plays an important role in studies of immune function, immune deficiency, effects of environmental factors, and comparative immunology. Applications for this technology have grown as the instruments have improved, with multiple lasers for exciting a wide range of fluorescent markers, improved fluidics, and increasingly useful software with modeling capabilities. Continued development of reagents for human and domestic species and studies of antibody cross-reactivity are advancing the capabilities of this technology for studies of exotic animals. Identification of laboratories with the expertise and equipment necessary for accurate analysis of samples and proper sample collection, handling, and transportation are key elements for successful flow cytometry studies.

References

[1] Kaleem Z. Flow cytometric analysis of lymphomas: current status and usefulness. Arch Pathol Lab Med 2006;130(12):1850–8.

[2] Weiss DJ. Application of flow cytometric techniques to veterinary clinical hematology. Vet Clin Pathol 2002;31(2):72–82.

[3] Byrne KM, Reinhart GA, Hayek MG. Standardized flow cytometry gating in veterinary medicine. Methods Cell Sci 2000;22(2–3):191–8.

[4] Byrne KM, Kim HW, Chew BP, et al. A standardized gating technique for the generation of flow cytometry data for normal canine and normal feline blood lymphocytes. Vet Immunol Immunopathol 2000;73(2):167–82.

[5] Zola H, Swart B, Nicholson I, et al. CD molecules 2005: human cell differentiation molecules. Blood 2005;106(9):3123–6.

[6] De Guise S, Erickson K, Blanchard M, et al. Characterization of a monoclonal antibody that recognizes a lymphocyte surface antigen for the cetacean homologue to CD45R. Immunology 1998;94(2):207–12.

[7] Bernier J, De Guise S, Martineau D, et al. Purification of functional T lymphocytes from splenocytes of the beluga whales (Delphinapterus leucas). Dev Comp Immunol 2000; 24(6–7):653–62.

[8] Schwartz J, Aldridge B, Blanchard M, et al. The development of methods for immunophenotypic and lymphocyte function analyses for assessment of Southern sea otter (Enhydra lutris nereis) health. Vet Immunol Immunopathol 2005;104(1–2):1–14.

[9] Available at: http://www.umass.edu/vetimm/. Accessed April 25, 2008.

[10] Saalmuller A, Aasted B. Summary of the animal homologue section of HLDA8. Vet Immunol Immunopathol 2007;119(1–2):2–13.

[11] DeLuca D, Wilson M, Warr GW. Lymphocyte heterogeneity in the trout, Salmo gairdneri, defined with monoclonal antibodies to IgM. Eur J Immunol 1983;13(7):546–51.

[12] Milston RH, Vella AT, Crippen TL, et al. In vitro detection of functional humoral immuno-competence in juvenile Chinook salmon (Oncorhynchus tshawytscha) using flow cytometry. Fish Shellfish Immunol 2003;15(2):145–58.

[13] Ronneseth A, Wergeland HI, Pettersen EF. Neutrophils and B-cells in Atlantic cod (Gadus morhua L.). Fish Shellfish Immunol 2007;23(3):493–503.

[14] Romano TA, Ridgway SH, Quaranta V. MHC class II molecules and immunoglobulins on peripheral blood lymphocytes of the bottlenosed dolphin, Tursiops truncatus. J Exp Zool 1992;263(1):96–104.

[15] Davis EG, Wilkerson MJ, Rush BR. Flow cytometry: clinical applications in equine medi-cine. J Vet Intern Med 2002;16(4):404–10.

[16] Wilkerson MJ, Shuman W, Swist S, et al. Platelet size, platelet surface-associated IgG, and reticulated platelets in dogs with immune-mediated thrombocytopenia. Vet Clin Pathol 2001;30(3):141–9.

[17] Mutinelli F, Vascellari M, Melchiotti E. Mediastinal lymphoma in a badger (Meles meles). J Wildl Dis 2004;40(1):129–32.

[18] Simmons HA, Fitzgerald SD, Kiupel M, et al. Multicentric T-cell lymphoma in a dromedary camel (Camelus dromedarius). J Zoo Wildl Med 2005;36(4):727–9.

[19] Wilkerson MJ, Dolce K, Koopman T, et al. Lineage differentiation of canine lymphoma/leu-kemias and aberrant expression of CD molecules. Vet Immunol Immunopathol 2005; 106(3–4):179–96.

[20] Vernau W, Moore PF. An immunophenotypic study of canine leukemias and preliminary assessment of clonality by polymerase chain reaction. Vet Immunol Immunopathol 1999; 69(2–4):145–64.

[21] English RV, Nelson P, Johnson CM, et al. Development of clinical disease in cats experimen-tally infected with feline immunodeficiency virus. J Infect Dis 1994;170(3):543–52.

[22] Novotney C, English RV, Housman J, et al. Lymphocyte population changes in cats naturally infected with feline immunodeficiency virus. AIDS 1990;4(12):1213–8.

[23] Torten M, Franchini M, Barlough JE, et al. Progressive immune dysfunction in cats experimentally infected with feline immunodeficiency virus. J Virol 1991;65(5):2225–30.

[24] Bull ME, Kennedy-Stoskopf S, Levine JF, et al. Evaluation of T lymphocytes in captive African lions (Panthera leo) infected with feline immunodeficiency virus. Am J Vet Res 2003;64(10):1293–300.

[25] Roelke ME, Pecon-Slattery J, Taylor S, et al. T-lymphocyte profiles in FIV-infected wild lions and pumas reveal CD4 depletion. J Wildl Dis 2006;42(2):234–48.

[26] Zhang S, Wood C, Xue W, et al. Immune suppression in calves with bovine immunodeficiency virus. Clin Diagn Lab Immunol 1997;4(2):232–5.

[27] Marodi L, Notarangelo LD. Immunological and genetic bases of new primary immunode-ficiencies. Nat Rev Immunol 2007;7(11):851–61.

[28] Felsburg PJ, Hartnett BJ, Henthorn PS, et al. Canine X-linked severe combined immunode-ficiency. Vet Immunol Immunopathol 1999;69(2–4):127–35.

[29] Perryman LE. Molecular pathology of severe combined immunodeficiency in mice, horses, and dogs. Vet Pathol 2004;41(2):95–100.

[30] Meek K, Kienker L, Dallas C, et al. SCID in Jack Russell terriers: a new animal model of DNA-PKcs deficiency. J Immunol 2001;167(4):2142–50.

[31] Wiler R, Leber R, Moore BB, et al. Equine severe combined immunodeficiency: a defect in V(D)J recombination and DNA-dependent protein kinase activity. Proc Natl Acad Sci U S A 1995;92(25):11485–9.

[32] Uchiyama R, Moritomo T, Kai O, et al. Counting absolute number of lymphocytes in quail whole blood by flow cytometry. J Vet Med Sci 2005;67(4):441–4.

[33] Martin RA, Brott DA, Zandee JC, et al. Differential analysis of animal bone marrow by flow cytometry. Cytometry 1992;13(6):638–43.

[34] Inoue T, Moritomo T, Tamura Y, et al. A new method for fish leucocyte counting and partial differentiation by flow cytometry. Fish Shellfish Immunol 2002;13(5):379–90.

[35] Waters WR, Palmer MV, Thacker TC, et al. Antigen-specific proliferation and activation of peripheral blood mononuclear cells from Mycobacterium bovis-infected reindeer. Vet Immunol Immunopathol 2006;111(3–4):263–77.

[36] Harford AJ, O'Halloran K, Wright PF. The effects of in vitro pesticide exposures on the phagocytic function of four native Australian freshwater fish. Aquat Toxicol 2005;75(4): 330–42.

[37] Harford AJ, O'Halloran K, Wright PE. Effect of in vitro and in vivo organotin exposures on the immune functions of Murray cod (Maccullochella peelii peelii). Environ Toxicol Chem 2007;26(8):1649–56.

[38] Utoh J, Harasaki H. Effects of temperature on phagocytosis of human and calf polymorpho-nuclear leukocytes. Artif Organs 1992;16(4):377–81.

[39] Harford AJ, O'Halloran K, Wright PF. Flow cytometric analysis and optimisation for measuring phagocytosis in three Australian freshwater fish. Fish Shellfish Immunol 2006; 20(4):562–73.

[40] Holloway J, Scheuhammer AM, Chan HM. Assessment of white blood cell phagocytosis as an immunological indicator of methylmercury exposure in birds. Arch Environ Contam Toxicol 2003;44(4):493–501.

[41] De Guise S, Erickson K, Blanchard M, et al. Characterization of F21.A, a monoclonal antibody that recognize a leucocyte surface antigen for killer whale homologue to beta-2 integrin. Vet Immunol Immunopathol 2004;97(3–4):195–206.

[42] DiMolfetto-Landon L, Erickson KL, Blanchard-Channell M, et al. Blastogenesis and inter-leukin-2 receptor expression assays in the harbor seal (Phoca vitulina). J Wildl Dis 1995; 31(2):150–8.

[43] Milovanova TN. Comparative analysis between CFSE flow cytometric and tritiated thymi-dine incorporation tests for beryllium sensitivity. Cytometry B Clin Cytom 2007;72(4): 265–75.

[44] Lyons AB, Parish CR. Determination of lymphocyte division by flow cytometry. J Immunol Methods 1994;171(1):131–7.

[45] Morrison RN, Lyons AB, Nowak BF, et al. Snapper (Pagrus auratus) leucocyte proliferation is synergistically enhanced by simultaneous stimulation with LPS and PHA. Fish Shellfish Immunol 2004;16(3):307–19.

[46] Schumacher A. Effect of ex vivo storage and Cyto-Chex on the expression of P-selectin glycoprotein ligand-1 (PSGL-1) on human peripheral leukocytes. J Immunol Methods 2007;323(1):24–30.

ELSEVIER SAUNDERS

Vet Clin Exot Anim 11 (2008) 597–609

VETERINARY
CLINICS
Exotic Animal Practice

Index

Note: Page numbers of article titles are in **boldface** type.

A

Abdominal vein, blood collection from, in amphibians, 465, 467
  in frogs and salamanders, 432

Abscesses, oral, hematologic disorders related to, in rabbits, 557

Activated partial thromboplastin time (APTT), in ferrets, 436

Adenocarcinomas, uterine, hematologic disorders related to, in rabbits, 556–557

Adrenal disease, ferret hematologic disorders and, 544, 548

Age, of amphibians, erythropoiesis differences based on, 474
    hematologic disorders related to, 464
  of ferrets, hemogram values based on, 542–543

Amphibians, blood collection techniques for, 464–468
    blood smear preparation, 468
    blood volume and, 464
    restraint for, 465–466
    sampling handling, 467–468
    venipuncture sites, 465–467
  hematologic disorders of, **463–480**
    bacterial infections causing, 476
    environmental factors in, 464
    fungal infections causing, 476
    hematopoiesis and, 474
    natural history of, 464
    neoplasia causing, 477
    normal cell morphology and function vs., 471–473
    parasitic infections causing, 476–477
    result interpretations for, 474–476
    summary overview of, 463–464
    test for, 468–471
    toxicants causing, 477–478
    viral infections causing, 476

Anaphylaxis, hematologic disorders related to, in avians, 513–514

Anatomic factors, of hematologic disorders, in amphibians, 464

Anemia, immune-mediated, flow cytometry detection of, 588
  in avians, clinical approach to, 506–508
    etiologies of, 504–507, 517
  in ferrets, 541
    estrous and, 544
  in fish, 450–451
    etiologies of, 452–453
    viral diseases and, 451, 453
  in potbellied pigs, 576–580
    etiologies of, 576, 578–579
    infectious diseases causing, 577, 580
    mineral deficiencies and, 576–577
    toxicities causing, 577
    vitamin deficiencies and, 576–577
  in rabbits, 554–555
  in reptiles, 494
  in rodents, 532
    bone marrow evaluation for, 530

Anesthetic agents, for blood collection, in amphibians, 465
    in ferrets, 535, 543
    in fish, 433–434
    in frogs, 431–432
    in giant spiders, 440–441
    in guinea pigs, 438
    in hedgehogs, 439
    in potbellied pigs, 569–570, 573
    in rodents, 524, 526
    in sugar gliders, 440
  for bone marrow collection, in rodents, 530–531

Anisocytosis, in avians, 503
  in rabbits, 553

Anterior vena cava, blood collection from, in potbellied pigs, 571

Moving?

Make sure your subscription moves with you!

To notify us of your new address, find your **Clinics Account Number** (located on your mailing label above your name), and contact customer service at:

E-mail: elspcs@elsevier.com

800-654-2452 (subscribers in the U.S. & Canada)
1-407-563-6020 (subscribers outside of the U.S. & Canada)

Fax number: 407-363-9661

Elsevier Periodicals Customer Service
6277 Sea Harbor Drive
Orlando, FL 32887-4800

*To ensure uninterrupted delivery of your subscription, please notify us at least 4 weeks in advance of move.